foundations of
massage
third edition

'health' — from the Old English *health*, meaning a state of wholeness,
and *haelan*, to heal or make whole

Dedicated to healers, past, present and future whose skills, knowledge and intent
assist to restore wholeness through the medium of touch.

foundations of massage
third edition

Lisa Casanelia
BHSc (MST), BA, RMT
Senior Lecturer — Remedial Therapies Dept, Endeavour College of
Natural Health, Melbourne, Australia

David Stelfox
Grad Dip Western Herb Med, BNat, Dip Rem Mass, Dip Nat,
Dip Herb Med
Academic Coordinator — Endeavour College of Natural Health,
Adelaide Campus
National Program Leader — Remedial Therapies Dept, Endeavour
College of Natural Health, Adelaide, Australia

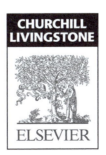

CHURCHILL
LIVINGSTONE

ELSEVIER

Sydney Edinburgh London New York Philadelphia St Louis Toronto

Churchill Livingstone
is an imprint of Elsevier

ELSEVIER

Elsevier Australia. ACN 001 002 357
(a division of Reed International Books Australia Pty Ltd)
Tower 1, 475 Victoria Avenue, Chatswood, NSW 2067

National Library of Australia Cataloguing-in-Publication Data

Casanelia, Lisa.

Foundations of massage / Lisa Casanelia; David Stelfox.

3rd ed.

9780729538695 (pbk.)

Includes index.
Bibliography.

Massage--Technique.
Massage--Philosophy.

Stelfox, David P.

615.822

Publisher: Sophie Kaliniecki
Developmental Editor: Sabrina Chew
Publishing Services Manager: Helena Klijn
Editorial Coordinator: Sarah Botros
Edited and indexed by Jon Forsyth
Proofread by Maria McGivern
Illustrations and internal design by Trina McDonald
Appendix illustrations by Nives Porcellato & Andrew Craig
Cover design by Stan Lamond
Photography by Glenn McCulloch Photography
Typeset by TNQ Books and Journals
Printed by Ligare

PEFC
PEFC/21-31-17

The book has been printed on paper certified
by the Programme for the Endorsement of
Forest Certification (PEFC). PEFC is
committed to sustainable forest management
through third party forest certification
of responsibly managed forests.

contents

foreword

'Massage is the study of anatomy in braille'
Jack Meagher

The sense of touch is one of our most underestimated of senses. Massage of course, is a celebration of the sense of touch and since ancient times this art has found practitioners in almost all cultures, who used it for relaxation, for therapy, for rehabilitation, and for remediation of health problems. Presently throughout the world, we are experiencing a resurgence of traditional, complementary and alternative modes of treatment. Massage, like the sense of touch, has always been a constant in the background, its practice uninterrupted during the passage of the centuries. However, we are now seeing massage coming to the forefront of health care in many areas.

Massage is being embraced in more and more situations of the modern world, an affirmation of its effectiveness throughout the centuries. Massage therapists can deliver effective treatments at gymnasiums, health clubs, private health care clinics and health spas. Corporate health care often incorporates massage and many sporting clubs have a massage practitioner on their payroll. Many massage therapists run their own practice, and increasingly remedial massage is standard care at many hospitals and aged-care facilities. Massage is nowadays very much 'mainstream', rather than 'alternative'.

The demand for competent, well-trained, professional massage practitioners requires a way of training and educating them to a national standard with well-defined benchmarks to relaxation and remedial skill sets. Although many massage courses exist around Australasia in a variety of training settings, many of these until recently use educational materials and texts that have been developed abroad. The success of the present text as a locally written resource is highlighted by this third edition you are now holding in your hands. Its rewriting, revision, updating and enhancement has assured it of a continuing valued place amongst Australasian schools that train massage practitioners.

This textbook is comprehensive and geared towards an Australasian audience in terms of cultural, ethical and legal considerations. Experienced massage practitioners, passionate educators and researchers have contributed to the textbook and the scientific basis of massage therapy is considered, while the latest research is incorporated into the practical aspects of massage that the book deals with. Clear, comprehensive text is complemented by relevant illustrative material that re-enforces the learning experience. Case-based approaches are enhanced by practical, clinical advice and supported by reference to industry-specific legislation. The appendixes and other additional reference material of the book further add to the usefulness of the text. Learning-oriented devices are incorporated into the book at many levels, making it student-friendly and a pleasure to use both from a teacher's as well as from a student's perspective.

I trust that you will find in this latest edition of *Foundations of Massage* an old friend rejuvenated and much improved. While many teachers and students of massage have benefitted from using its predecessors, the current edition will make new friends and help in the training of competent, informed, well-rounded massage practitioners.

Dr Nicholas J. Vardaxis
Director of Education,
Endeavour College of Natural Health,
Melbourne 2009

preface

The resurgence and growth of interest in personal health and wellbeing that emerged in the last decades of the twentieth century is very apparent in the increased demand these days for services in the areas of fitness, beauty and natural health care. Of all the modalities or areas of natural health, massage therapy is perhaps the most commonly accepted and utilised. Once regarded as a luxury, massage therapy is now regarded by many as an essential means for promoting and maintaining optimum health, fitness and wellbeing. In a stressed-out world, where individuals feel increasingly isolated and deprived of touch, relaxation massage provides welcome relief, and is an important and effective therapy, of benefit to a wide range of people and conditions.

The increased demand for massage therapy by consumers has resulted in the need for competently trained massage therapists and in the establishment of national standards of education and training for massage therapy practice. In Australia and New Zealand, government-accredited health training packages have instituted benchmarks of education standards for a number of natural health care modalities, including relaxation massage and remedial massage therapy. Additionally, national peak bodies and professional associations for natural medicine and massage therapy ensure that the standard of practice provided by practitioners is consistent and high.

With the introduction of these education standards, it became apparent that the only massage therapy texts available were overseas publications, and that there was an urgent need for a comprehensive text that presented the fundamentals of massage therapy from a uniquely Australian perspective. The first edition of *Foundations of Massage* succeeded in satisfying this need. It became the text of choice for providers of massage therapy education throughout Australia. For the second edition we brought together an experienced team of practitioners and educators to expand the scope of the text. The inclusion of additional chapters covering areas such as infection control, pharmacological considerations and self-care ensured that all aspects of massage therapy practice were covered comprehensively and appropriately. Not only was the second edition taken up by more schools and colleges in Australia, but it also gained popularity as a massage text in New Zealand.

In this, the third edition of *Foundations of Massage,* we have once again drawn together the knowledge and experience of massage therapists, health practitioners and health educators, not only from within Australia but also internationally, to provide an up-to-date, clinically based and well-rounded perspective on the practice of massage. These contributors possess not just a wealth of knowledge and experience, but also a passion for massage therapy and the benefits it can offer. It is our hope that this passion may rub off on the reader and student of this text and, along with the knowledge and skills outlined throughout, provide a strong foundation for effective and successful massage therapy practice. We trust that you will find this book informative, practical and enjoyable.

Lisa Casanelia
David Stelfox

acknowledgements

We wish to express our heart-felt thanks to the book's contributors, without whom this third edition would not have been possible. Thank you for sharing our vision for this text, and also for sharing your knowledge, expertise and passion for the art and science of massage. Our gratitude to Sophie Kaliniecki, Sabrina Chew, Helena Klijn and Sarah Botros from Elsevier Australia for their commitment to getting this edition to print on time.

Thanks also to the reviewers who provided feedback which assisted with the update of this text.

Finally we wish to acknowledge those who initiated and contributed to the original idea for this foundation massage text. You know who you are. It was your vision, your motivation, your dedication and support that has resulted in the evolution of Foundations of Massage to this third edition.

reviewers

Paula Nutting, BHSc MST, Dip Rem Mass, Past Registered Nurse
National President, Australian Association of Massage Therapists

Allan Hudson, DRM, Dip Acup. Adv.Dip Nat
Faculty Head of Tactile Therapies and the School of Continuing Education, Nature Care College, Sydney, Australia

Diana L Thompson, LMP (licensed massage therapist)
President, Massage Therapy Foundation, Evanston, Illinois, USA

Carolyn Price, Dip Teaching, Cert IV TAA (Training and Assessment)
Cert IV Mass Ther, Dip Aroma, Reg.Teacher IAAMA (International Aromatherapy and Aromatic Medicine Association); Coordinator, Complementary Health Program, TAFE SA North, Adelaide, Australia

Jason Patten, M.ExcSci, Dip RM
Senior Educator, RMIT University, School of Life and Physical Sciences, College of Science, Engineering and Health, Melbourne, Australia

Choong Ng, MBBS BMedSci DipRM CertIVFitness
General Medical Practitioner, Evidence-Based Practice Researcher, Remedial Massage Therapist and Fitness Trainer (Private), Melbourne, Australia

Antony Porcino, BSc, CHP, PhD Candidate
Project Director, Complementary Medicine Education & Outcomes, BC Cancer Agency, Vancouver, Canada

Steve Lawson, MEd, BSc(CompMed),AdvDIpNat,Grad DipMFR,GradDipCST,DTS,DRM
Director of Education, Nature Care College, Sydney, Australia

contributors

David Stelfox, Grad Dip Western Herb Med, BNat, Dip Rem Mass, Dip Nat, Dip Herb Med
Academic Coordinator, Endeavour College of Natural Health, Adelaide Campus; National Program Leader — Remedial Therapies Dept, Endeavour College of Natural Health, Adelaide, Australia

Katharine Callaway, BHSc (Natural Medicine), Dip App Sc (RemTh)

Susan Burgess, Dip HSc (Remedial Therapies), Dip (Reflexology) Dip (Indian Head Mass) LST
Remedial Massage and Reflexology practitioner, Denmark

Sheena Worrall, Grad Cert Higher Education, Dip Ther Mass
Lecturer, Faculties of Social Science and Bioscience, Endeavour College of Natural Health, Gold Coast, Australia

Janine Tobin, BHMS, BN, Dip Remedial Massage, Grad Cert Higher Education
Lecturer, Faculty of Biosciences, Endeavour College of Natural Health, Brisbane, Australia

Sonya Bailey, Grad Cert Higher Education, BHSc (MST)
Lecturer, Faculty of Remedial Therapies, Endeavour College of Natural Health, Melbourne, Australia

Sandra Grace, PhD, MSc Chiro (Res), Grad Cert Sports Chiro, Dip Acup, DBM, DC, DO, Dip Ed
BA Research Fellow, The Education for Practice Institute, Charles Sturt University, Australia

Lisa Casanelia, BHSc (MST), BA, RMT
Senior Lecturer — Remedial Therapies Dept, Endeavour College of Natural Health, Melbourne, Australia

Ellie Feeney, BHSc (MST), DipAppSc (RemTh), RN, RM
Senior Lecturer — Bioscience Dept, Endeavour College of Natural Health, Melbourne, Australia

Heather Morrison, PhD, BSc (Hons)
Head of School — Health Science, Endeavour College of Natural Health, Melbourne, Australia

Jan Douglass, BHSc, Dip Rem Mass
Lymphoedema Therapist, Flinders Surgical Oncology Clinic, Flinders Medical Centre, Adelaide Australia; Instructor, Vodder Schools International
Michael Nott, BScHons (Melbourne), PhD (Strathclyde)
Senior Lecturer, Discipline of Pharmaceutical Sciences, RMIT University, Melbourne, Australia

Lauriann Greene, CEAS
Co-author, *Save Your Hands! The Complete Guide to Injury Prevention and Ergonomics for Manual Therapists,* 2nd edn

Richard W Goggins, M.S., CPE, LMP
Co-author, *Save Your Hands! The Complete Guide to Injury Prevention and Ergonomics for Manual Therapists,* 2nd edn

Steven Goldstein, BA (Education), BHSc.(MST)
Education Chair, Australian Association Massage Therapists; Senior Lecturer, Faculty of Remedial Therapies, Endeavour College of Natural Health, Melbourne, Australia

Margaret (Margo) Hutchison, RN, Dip IYTA, Dip Ther Mass, Grad Cert Higher Education
On-line Course Tutor, Sessional Lecturer — Bio-Science Dept, Endeavour College of Natural Health, Brisbane, Australia

Suzanne Yates, BA (Hons), DipHSEC, MRSS(T), APNT, PGCE
Body-worker and birth educator, Director of Well Mother, Bristol, England

Clare Thorp, RN, GradDip (Public Health), GradDip (Health Education), Dip (Aromatherapy, Cert Mass Ther, Cert IV Reflex
Practitioner Trainer and Certified Infant Massage Instructor, Infant Massage Australia

philosophies and principles of massage and natural medicine
David Stelfox

chapter 1

LEARNING OUTCOMES

- **Define massage**
- **Describe the philosophies, principles and practice of massage therapy within the context of natural medicine**
- **Define and provide examples of complementary and alternative health care therapies**
- **Compare and contrast the principles and practices of chiropractic, osteopathy, physiotherapy and massage therapy**

INTRODUCTION

To be a competent and successful massage therapist — or, for that matter, a health professional of any modality — a clear understanding of the nature (definition) of the discipline, as well as its guiding philosophy and principles, is essential. Without such understanding a health care practitioner cannot deliver consistent therapeutic services that lie within a clearly defined scope of practice. It is a bit like having a car without a road map to help you find your way.

Massage therapy is generally classified as a 'complementary' or 'alternative' form of health care and is generally perceived to be one of many modalities which come under the classification of 'Natural Medicine' (House of Lords Report 2000). These are terms that also require definition and understanding. This chapter aims at providing the massage student with an understanding of the various philosophies, principles and definitions associated with natural medicine practice. Through this understanding the student should feel that they have an orientation to the profession in which they will be practicing.

MASSAGE THERAPY — A DEFINITION

One of the difficulties of defining massage is that the term means many things to many people. The terms massage, tactile therapy, bodywork, manual therapy and manipulative therapy have different connotations and different interpretations.

Massage as a profession has evolved significantly over the last century and today many different styles, techniques and approaches are embraced by the term 'massage'. There are now so many different techniques and approaches to soft tissue manipulation that it is difficult to classify them clearly under meaningful categories. Many have tried, but confusion has often resulted, as there will always be techniques that don't fit neatly under the proposed categories. For the purpose of this text, the more commonly known methods are classified under three broad headings — the subtle energy practices, the relaxation methods, and the remedial approaches (see Table 1.1).

For the purpose of defining massage, the historical roots of the word 'massage', and their individual meanings, will be examined. 'Massage' means to touch, softly press, squeeze, rub, handle or knead with the hands. The English word 'massage' first appeared in American and European literature around 1875. It was popularised in the USA by Douglas Graham from Massachusetts (who wrote a history of the art) and in Europe by an influential Dutchman, Dr Johann Mezger.

The Greek word *masso* or *massein* means to touch, handle, knead or squeeze. *Massa* is the Latin root coming directly from the Greek, and is reflected in the Portuguese verb *amassar*, to knead. The Arabic root *mass'h*, or *mass*, is very similar and means to press softly, as does the Sanskrit *makeh*. Ancient Jewish culture held the power of touch for ritual benefit in such high esteem that the root word for anointing and rubbing with oils and for the Messiah is the same (Mãshiãh).

Massage is usually applied to the skin, fascia, muscles, tendons and ligaments (the soft tissues) of the body. Since most massage has the effect of bringing about some sort of positive change in the individual,

Table 1.1 Categories of massage therapy

Subtle energy practices	Relaxation methods	Remedial approaches
Reiki	Swedish massage	Manual lymphatic drainage
Therapeutic touch	Esalen massage	Neuromuscular technique
Polarity therapy		Myofascial release
Pranic healing		Aromatherapy
Aura balancing		Reflexology
Chakra balancing		An mo tui na (Chinese massage)
Jin shin do		Shiatsu
Zero balancing		Muscle energy technique
		Rolfing
		Postural integration
		Bowen technique
		Orthobionomy
		Craniosacral therapy
		Trager therapy
		Sports massage

then its action may be said to be therapeutic in that it provides physical, emotional, psychological or spiritual benefits. Therefore, the term 'therapeutic massage' applies to all methods and forms of massage, since they all provide therapeutic benefit to the receiver. Reduction of muscular tension, improvement of vascular and lymphatic circulation, regulation of the nervous system and normalisation of pulmonary function are some of the claimed therapeutic physiological benefits of massage therapy (Turchaninov 2001).

Massage therapy, then, may be defined as the use of (predominantly) the hands to physically manipulate the body's soft tissues for the purpose of effecting a desirable change in the individual. While anatomical and physiological changes are generally the focus, and may involve body systems other than the musculoskeletal system, the emotional, mental and spiritual aspects of the individual may also be affected, either objectively or subjectively due to their interrelatedness. Typical fundamental massage techniques involve, but are not necessarily restricted to, basic contact (touch), stroking (effleurage), rubbing (friction), kneading (pétrissage), percussion (tapôtement), vibration and compression. Usually a lubricant, such as an oil or powder is used. However, massage can also be provided without the use of a lubricant (i.e. dry massage), and may be given through clothing. Hot or cold applications (thermotherapy), essential (aromatic) oils or water (hydrotherapy) may be utilised as adjuncts to massage treatment where they are considered appropriate to providing the desired therapeutic effect.

Relaxation massage seeks to relax the client, improve general wellbeing and reduce mental stress and general body tension. Techniques employed aim to soothe and loosen the body. The speed of delivery is slow and the pressure is light to moderate. An environment is created which may include soft lighting to soothe the eyes, pictures and props to create further visual pleasure, and aromatic oils dispersed in the air to satisfy the mood and emotions. Music may be played to relax the mind and enhance the spirit, and the massage table is draped for comfort and warmth. The massage environment may contribute significantly to the outcome of enhanced wellbeing and relaxation experienced by the client. (See Chapter 8 for further discussion on the massage setting.)

Remedial massage is the application of more advanced techniques of treatment and assessment for neuro-musculoskeletal dysfunctions. The primary aim of remedial massage is to restore or promote motion and to reduce or prevent pain. To achieve this a variety of techniques may be employed. These may include thermotherapy, myofascial release techniques, neuromuscular techniques (trigger-point therapy), muscle energy techniques, joint mobilisation, positional release techniques, post-isometric stretching and corrective exercise prescription.

NATURAL MEDICINE PHILOSOPHY AND PRINCIPLES

The philosophical basis of massage therapy draws from the philosophy and principles of natural medicine in general. The field of natural medicine embraces many different individual modalities of natural therapies, including massage, homoeopathy, aromatherapy, osteopathy, colour therapy as well as complete systems of natural healing, such as traditional Chinese medicine, ayurveda, and naturopathy (House of Lords Report

2000). What draws these many different approaches together under the one umbrella is the philosophy that provides guidelines to their practice.

Natural medicine is most simply defined as *any form of health care that acknowledges and relies upon the body's natural ability to heal itself*. This principle has been a feature of traditional medicine practices for thousands of years. Traditional medicine is a term used to describe any system of health care that has ancient roots, trained healers, cultural bonds and a theoretical construct; for example, traditional Chinese medicine, ayurveda, herbal medicine (Segen 1998). Natural medicine philosophy acknowledges nature's ability to heal *(vis medicatrix naturae — the healing power of nature)*. Given the right circumstances (e.g. rest, nurturing, living according to nature's laws) a sick or injured individual can return naturally to a state of optimum health. This can be easily illustrated by the example of a fractured bone. Over a period of time the bone will heal (i.e. become whole again) of its own accord. It requires no intervention, although immobilisation may assist the bone to return to its original shape. *The body heals itself*, and nature provides the body with this ability. Any form of therapy, whether massage, nutrition, acupuncture, herbs or surgery, works simply by assisting nature's own ability to heal.

Apart from this core principle of the body's ability to heal itself, there are a number of other principles which feature commonly in natural medicine modalities and these are discussed below.

Treat the whole person

Optimum health and wellbeing is a complex interrelationship between the physical, mental, emotional and spiritual aspects of an individual (see Chapter 3). When imbalance occurs on any of these levels it eventually results in disease. For example, long-term emotional stress will eventually affect the physical body via the nervous and endocrine systems. It can then manifest physically as muscle tension, neck and back pain, headache and physical fatigue. On the physical level, natural medicine acknowledges and addresses the interrelationship between every cell, tissue, organ and system of the body. Injury or illness is never seen to be affecting just an isolated part of the body. A change to one part results in change to every part. Since illness can be the result of an imbalance in any, or a combination, of these aspects then healing must address each of them. Tactile therapy, including massage, has the potential to impact upon every aspect of the individual and so it treats the whole person.

First do no harm

Natural medicine uses therapies which are as close as possible to their natural state (e.g. human touch, herbs, food and nutrition) and that are unlikely to produce harmful side effects. Practitioners of natural medicine, including massage therapists, learn to assess the health of clients and determine whether they can effectively treat them, or if referral to another health care practitioner is more appropriate.

Prevention is better than cure

Wherever possible, the practitioner of natural medicine will promote a strategy that helps to prevent illness from eventuating, or at least from becoming worse, in the case of existing ailments. This is achieved via a combination of treatments and by involving clients in the process (e.g. regular exercise, adequate rest, balanced diet). Regular massage can serve the purpose of relaxing the nervous system, toning or relaxing muscles and regulating circulation of body fluids, thereby promoting optimum health and reducing the risk of illness or injury.

The doctor (practitioner) is a teacher

The original meaning of the word 'doctor' was 'teacher'. To achieve the best treatment outcome, to prevent the onset of illness or injury and to maintain optimum health and wellbeing, the natural medicine practitioner must educate her/his clients to take responsibility for their wellness and to get involved with creating their own health. Only by encouraging clients to live a more balanced lifestyle according to nature's laws, including healthy dietary choices, regular exercise or activity, and adequate rest, can the practitioner hope to assist. By teaching, motivating and supporting clients the practitioner–client relationship is empowered. This relationship in itself contributes significantly to the process of healing (Pizzorno & Murray 1999).

The World Health Organization (WHO) estimates that 80% of the world's population utilises natural medicine as its primary source of health care (WHO 1998). In Australia, around 69% of the population uses natural medicine of some kind (Pfizer Australia Health Report 2006). These Australians are more likely to be female, aged 30–50 years, have tertiary qualifications, earn more than $50 000 per year and be employed in a professional or managerial position. They choose natural medicine because they are dissatisfied with other approaches to health care, and because they see it as a natural, safe alternative (Therapeutic Goods Administration 2001). In view of these facts then, natural medicine can hardly be seen as a radical, alternative healing approach on the fringe of the mainstream biomedical model of health care. With well over half of the population relying upon it to achieve a desired level of health, it is not unreasonable to view natural medicine as part of 'mainstream medicine'.

COMPLEMENTARY AND ALTERNATIVE MEDICINE

Natural medicine is sometimes referred to as 'complementary and alternative medicine' (CAM). Alternative medicine is a term that was used more commonly during the 1980s and early 1990s. *The New England*

Journal of Medicine (1992: 61) defined alternative medicine as:

> ... a heterogeneous set of practices that are offered as an alternative to conventional medicine, for the preservation of health and the diagnosis and treatment of health-related problems; its practitioners are often called healers.

At the time, this explanation reflected the fact that a minority of the population of the Western world used natural therapies as an alternative to mainstream Western biomedicine. 'Alternative' suggests an either/or choice, and provides no suggestion that Western biomedicine and natural medicine could possibly work together for the ultimate benefit of clients. Alternative medicine, then, is something which is used as an alternative to (i.e. to the exclusion of) conventional mainstream medicine approaches. These days, the natural medicine profession generally rejects the term 'alternative', as it prefers to view itself as part of an integrated approach to health care (see Chapter 3).

By definition, the term 'complementary' means to form a satisfactory or balanced whole (*Collins Concise Dictionary* 1989). When used to describe natural medicine, 'complementary' suggests that in conjunction with the Western biomedical approach to health care, the two form a satisfactory and balanced holistic health care model (i.e. an integrated approach). However, it is taken by some to suggest that natural medicine plays only a secondary role to the biomedical model, providing merely a supplementary approach where appropriate, and cannot provide a stand-alone option to the management of health. In this respect, the term 'complementary' is an unsatisfactory description of natural medicine. Another perspective is that complementary medicine is something which may be used to enhance, but not to replace, a conventional mainstream approach to the treatment of a health condition.

SCOPE OF PRACTICE OF NATURAL MEDICINE MODALITIES

The philosophy and principles of natural medicine define and guide the practice of the many therapies that comprise this approach to health care. Most have unique knowledge bases (i.e. the theory and skills that define how the therapy is administered), although there is some overlap (e.g. Chinese massage and acupuncture with their philosophy of Qi and energy flow through meridians or channels). As a result, the scope of practice (see Chapter 5) of these natural medicine modalities often overlaps, and is not always clear or definite. It is important for massage therapists to have a basic understanding of other natural medicine modalities and their scopes of practice. The following is a brief outline of some of the more common natural medicine modalities.

Acupuncture and traditional Chinese medicine

Acupuncture involves the insertion of fine needles, and the application of a burning herb material known as moxa, to very specific points or areas on the body. It is a therapy practised as part of the traditional Chinese medicine (TCM) system, which is based on the Chinese philosophical concept of health and disease. This philosophy states that health is promoted and maintained via the unobstructed flow of vital energy referred to as Qi through subtle channels that run throughout the body. Illness occurs when the flow of Qi becomes obstructed. Diagnosis is achieved via thorough case taking, and pulse and tongue analysis. Acupuncture and moxibustion (i.e. the burning of moxa) when administered to points located on these channels (meridians) restore and regulate the flow of Qi. The TCM system also incorporates Chinese massage (an mo tui na), Chinese herbal medicine, diet and food therapy and exercise therapy (e.g. tai qi, qi gong). While some practitioners of Chinese medicine may include all of these therapies in their practice, others may specialise in only some or even one (e.g. acupuncture or Chinese herbs).

Aromatherapy

Aromatherapy involves the administration of essential oils distilled from plants to treat and prevent illness and to promote wellbeing. The oils may be administered topically through the dermal interface, via massage, compress, poultice, creams and ointments, through the respiratory interface by means of a variety of inhalation techniques or less commonly via the digestive interface through internal ingestion. An extensive range of health conditions may be treated with aromatherapy. Most aromatherapists are trained in basic relaxation massage and, more often than not, also in the technique of specialised aromatherapy massage such as that developed by Marguerite Maury (2004), an Austrian born biochemist who significantly influenced modern aromatherapy practice.

Ayurveda

Ayurveda is a traditional system of healing originating from the Indian subcontinent. It is thought to be the oldest existing system of medicine practiced in the world. Ayurveda has its own unique principles based primarily on the three doshas (physiology/personality types). Pulse, tongue and urine analysis form part of the method for diagnosis. Therapies used include herbal medicine, diet and nutrition, massage, colour therapy, exercise (yoga), meditation, sound therapy, lifestyle counselling and aromatherapy. In the West, ayurveda has become increasingly popular due largely to the writings of Indian-born endocrinologist Dr Deepak Chopra (author of *Creating Health*, *Perfect Health*, *Quantum Healing* and other texts).

Herbal medicine

Herbal medicine practitioners usually specialise in the use of plant medicines (herbs) to treat any of a wide variety of health conditions. While naturopaths usually incorporate herbs as part of their treatment strategy, along with nutrition, massage, flower essences and perhaps homoeopathy, the herbalist will generally prescribe only herbal remedies. Phytotherapy and botanical medicine are terms also used as alternatives to 'herbal medicine'. Herbal remedies were one of the earliest forms of medication used by humankind, and most traditional healing systems include them as part of their treatment of ill health.

Homoeopathy

By comparison with ayurveda, traditional Chinese medicine and even naturopathy, homoeopathy is a relative newcomer to the field of natural medicine. It originated in Germany in the 1830s as the result of investigation by Dr Samuel Hahnemann. Based on the principle of 'like cures like' (*similia similibus curantur*), the concept of homoeopathy is that a substance that can cause illness could also cure that same illness when administered in greatly diluted doses (e.g. arsenic). Despite numerous controlled trials indicating benefits for the treatment of a wide number of health problems, homoeopathy defies explanation in terms of its mechanism of cure. Scientists have failed to provide an explanation of how something that contains virtually no physical substance apart from water can demonstrate an efficacy comparable with, and even better than, that of pharmaceutical drugs.

Classical homoeopaths seek to establish the single best homoeopathic remedy to suit clients' presenting signs and symptoms, and prescribe no other form of therapy or remedy. However, many naturopaths incorporate homoeopathic remedies in their treatment strategy for clients when they consider them to be appropriate.

Naturopathy

The term 'naturopathy' was first used in 1899, in the USA. It was an approach to health care based on the principles of 'nature cure' from Europe. Nature cure was a general term used throughout Europe during the nineteenth century to describe the use of natural principles and therapies to prevent and treat disease. However, naturopathy's roots go back to ancient Greece and the 'father of medicine', Hippocrates, who believed that 'nature is the healer of all disease'. Disease was viewed as a result of violation of nature's laws, and fresh air, pure water, whole foods, sunlight, exercise and adequate rest and relaxation are seen as the cornerstones of healthy living.

In addition to promoting these healthy lifestyle measures, naturopathic practice integrates a number of modalities, principally nutrition, herbal medicine and tactile therapy. Other modalities, such as homoeopathy, aromatherapy, flower essence therapy, applied kinesiology, and hydrotherapy may also be incorporated. These modalities are applied on the basis of specific principles, and within the context of a healing environment, which endeavours to empower the individual, and motivate and educate them in order to restore, maintain and optimise wellbeing. By way of in-depth consultations, naturopaths decide upon strategies of treatment that will incorporate the most appropriate remedy/remedies to suit clients and their individual health condition. The health assessment may also be aided by naturopathic diagnostic methods such as iris, tongue and fingernail analysis, and also by physical examination and pathology tests.

Nutrition therapy

Nutrition therapy, nutritional medicine, or clinical nutrition as it is also known, incorporates dietary counselling (i.e. recommending appropriate changes to clients' diets), food therapy (i.e. foods with therapeutic properties) and nutrient supplementation to treat any of a wide variety of health conditions. Supplementation with vitamins, minerals or other micronutrients is prescribed, not just where there may be deficiencies, but where an illness or injury has caused an increased demand for certain nutrients by the body. Clinical nutritionists are generally also trained in sports nutrition, an area that focuses on improving sporting performance and recovery via an optimum diet and nutrient supplementation where necessary. Treatment and management of allergies is another area in which nutrition therapists are usually trained. Where naturopaths usually incorporate diet and nutrition therapy as one of their therapeutic tools, along with herbs, massage, lifestyle counselling and sometimes homoeopathy, clinical nutritionists generally treat health problems exclusively with diet and nutrition therapy.

Tactile therapies

The field of tactile therapy includes an ever-increasing range of therapies that involve tactile manipulation (i.e. the use of touch). It is sometimes referred to as bodywork or physical therapy. While some forms of tactile therapy mainly promote beneficial changes to the anatomy and physiology of the physical body (e.g. relaxation, tonification, or stimulation of muscles, tendons, ligaments, nerves and circulation), others exert their effects mainly on the subtle anatomy/subtle energy of individuals. Reiki, therapeutic touch, aura massage and pranic healing are examples of tactile therapies that focus on changing the subtle energy/subtle body of clients. Although therapies such as Swedish massage, Chinese massage (an mo tui na), chiropractic, osteopathy, sports massage and rolfing exert their effects mainly on the physical body, it is insisted by some that they also have an effect on the subtle energy of clients (Tappan 1988; Chaitow 1996).

Because there are so many approaches to tactile therapy, it is inevitable that there are many similarities between them. This includes both similarity of technique and similarity in what they can achieve therapeutically. What they share in common exceeds how they differ. For this reason there is a lot of crossover when it comes to mapping the scope of practice of these different tactile therapy approaches. While most practitioners of tactile therapy are specialists in this particular area of natural medicine, others may incorporate tactile therapy as part of their overall approach to health care (e.g. with nutrition, acupuncture, herbal medicine, flower essences). Naturopaths are an example of this.

Eastern/Asian massage therapies

Oriental bodywork techniques are based on a different set of principles and philosophy than the Western approaches to massage. The various Eastern approaches

---

Box 1.1 Eastern/Asian bodywork approaches

- Acupressure
- An mo tui na (Chinese massage)
- Shiatsu (Japanese bodywork)
- Thai massage
- Balinese massage

(see Box 1.1) to bodywork use different techniques and approaches, but their purpose is similar. Basically all these approaches to bodywork aim to restore, balance or maintain the flow of Qi (vital force) throughout the body (see the sections on acupuncture and traditional Chinese medicine earlier in this chapter). It is the uninterrupted and harmonious flow of Qi that is responsible for maintaining physical, mental, emotional and spiritual health. When Qi is blocked, discomfort may be experienced spiritually, emotionally, mentally or physically. If this blockage persists over time, the imbalance develops in its complexity and eventually chronic and degenerative health conditions will result.

MANIPULATIVE THERAPIES

These days the term 'manipulative therapy' is used mainly to describe the practices of chiropractic, osteopathy and physiotherapy. The goal of manipulative therapy has been defined as 'to restore maximal, pain-free movement of the musculoskeletal system in postural balance' (Dvorak, Dvorak & Schneider 1985). This somewhat comprehensive definition was determined by 35 experts in the field of manipulative therapy at a workshop in Switzerland in 1983. By this widely accepted definition, massage therapy also qualifies as a form of manipulative therapy, but there are similarities and differences between them.

Manipulation therapy, like massage and other forms of tactile therapy, has been a part of the art and science of healing for thousands of years. Nearly every culture has had practitioners who specialised in bonesetting, vertebral adjustment and manipulation of tendons, fascia, ligaments and muscles (for example, ancient Egypt, Greece, Africa, North and South America, India and Asia). Bonesetters practised the art of precise hand thrusts to align the spinal vertebrae and also set and promote the healing of fractured bones. They have always been popular in rural areas, where farmers and manual labourers have sought their services.

History records camel drivers in Arabia who practised manipulation on each other, English peasant women who relieved others of back pain, young girls who were taught to walk on backs, and families of bonesetters who travelled from village to village practising their special art. These skills were often considered to be a special gift handed down from generation to generation (Kaptchuk & Croucher 1986). During the Middle Ages the clicking of a spinal joint that resulted from a physical manipulation was thought to be the expulsion of demons or spirits from the body. The presence of manipulative therapy has always been of importance in society, even though at times its popularity has declined, usually as a result of criticism or discouragement by religious bodies or biomedical practitioners. One such decline corresponded to (Greenman 1996: 3):

> ... the approximate time of the split of physicians and barber-surgeons. As physicians became less involved in patient contact and as direct hands-on patient care became the province of the barber-surgeons, the role of manual medicine in the healing art seems to have declined.

However, manipulative therapy has always risen again out of such declines. The most recent renaissance took place in the late nineteenth century, a period of turmoil and conflicting views in the field of medicine. At about the same time two gifted Americans, Andrew Taylor Still (1828–1917) and Daniel David Palmer (1845–1913) developed the systems of osteopathy and chiropractic respectively.

Osteopathy

Andrew Taylor Still developed osteopathy as an alternative to the existing practice of medicine of the time. Disenchanted with the heroic approach to medicine which included blood-letting, purging and heavy-handed prescribing of laxatives, calomel (mercury), narcotics and other drugs, Still developed his new 'osteopathic medicine' on a philosophy of traditional (i.e. longstanding) healing principles combined with a contemporary understanding of the functioning of the body. He began offering his new approach to the public in 1874. Manipulation therapy was added to his approach by 1879. Today manipulative therapy is the core of osteopathic practice. For some osteopaths, manipulation is the only therapy practised.

The philosophy of osteopathy is based on five key principles as follows:

1 The body is a unit — the body does not function as separate parts. All parts, including cells, tissues, organs, and body systems, relate to each other and function as an integrated unit. There is no hierarchy of parts (i.e. no one structure of the body is of greater importance than another). For optimum health to exist, all aspects of the body must function optimally and harmoniously.

2 The healing power of nature — the body has an innate capacity to heal and maintain health. The therapist's role is to support this capacity.

3 Structure and function are interrelated — when the structure of any body part is negatively affected, the function of that part, and other parts as well, will eventually be affected too. Conversely, if function is disturbed (e.g. through a nutrient deficiency), sooner or later the structure of the cells, tissues, organs or body systems will also be altered in some way.

4 When normal adaptability is disrupted, or when environmental changes overcome the body's capacity for self-maintenance, ill-health may follow — apart from the obvious, this also implies that the

therapist must always look for the cause/s of illness and address them appropriately. It is never enough simply to treat the illness or its signs and symptoms.

5 Rational treatment is based on all of the previous principles — in any dysfunction, in any illness, the function and/or structure, and eventually both, will be affected. The body attempts to self-correct via its inherent self-healing mechanism. If or when the body's capacity for self-maintenance and adaptation is overcome, signs and symptoms will manifest. The role of a good therapist is not just to relieve the symptoms, but to recognise the cause/s and how the body is attempting to cope with the situation. Having established this, the appropriate treatment is one which supports, promotes and enhances the body's potential for self-healing.

It is worth noting that these osteopathic principles outlined above are in keeping with those that form the basis of natural medicine philosophy as described earlier in this chapter.

In the USA, its country of origin, osteopathy has always been a total medical approach. Students of osteopathy in that country learn surgery and how to prescribe pharmaceutical drugs, along with structural assessment and diagnosis, and manipulative therapy skills. Taught within a framework of the philosophic principles established by Still, osteopathy may be said to offer total patient care and is a licensed health care profession throughout the US. However, in Australia, New Zealand and the UK, osteopathic training and practice is restricted to the skills and practice of physical manipulation, although Still's philosophy and principles are usually espoused as guidelines to osteopathic practice.

Techniques of osteopathic manipulation

Osteopathic manipulations are applied to both the soft tissues of the body, such as the muscles, ligaments, tendons, and fascia, and also to the bones and joints of the body. The aim of osteopathic manipulation is to achieve improved physiological movement, relief of pain or discomfort, relaxation of tissues, and to support the body's self-healing capacity. It is possible to classify osteopathic manipulative techniques into two broad categories — direct and indirect. Direct technique is that which confronts any restriction of movement by applying force to the body part in the direction of the restriction. With indirect technique the body part is manipulated in the direction of ease of motion. The physiological effects of a manipulation include changes to muscular tone, central, peripheral or autonomic nervous system tone, and circulatory system (lymphatic, vascular) response changes (Gallagher & Humphrey 2001).

Osteopaths may incorporate a variety of different specific techniques. Some of these include: high velocity, low amplitude (HVLA) thrusting; articulatory technique; soft tissue therapy (similar to massage); craniosacral technique; muscle energy technique; myofascial release; visceral stretching and balancing technique; and counter-strain technique.

An osteopathic treatment commences with the taking of a client's history, a physical examination of either the whole body or the region where the problem is located, possibly evaluation of X-rays, and the treatment itself. During the physical examination the osteopath seeks to identify the area/s of dysfunction in the musculoskeletal system. Having identified the problem and evaluated the cause/s, the therapist then determines the most appropriate manipulative technique and the degree of force required to achieve the desired result. Osteopaths generally use the least amount of force necessary. Follow-up treatments are determined on the basis of the client's response to the initial manipulation.

Chiropractic

Daniel David Palmer, the originator of chiropractic, was a magnetic healer and self-taught manipulative therapist from the US mid-west. Palmer developed the system of chiropractic ('done by hand') manipulative therapy in the 1890s, around the same time that Still developed osteopathy. While Palmer was chiropractic's originator, it was his son, Bartlett Joshua Palmer, who promoted the practice of this therapy to a professional status with a devoted following.

Chiropractic is based on four main principles:

1 The nervous system plays an important role in health and disease — the nervous system in human beings is highly developed and influences all other systems of the body, and their organs, tissues and cells.

2 The human body has the innate capacity to heal itself (*vis medicatrix naturae*) — chiropractic is based on the vitalistic theory which states that all living things are pervaded by a vital force, which maintains, promotes and restores health.

3 Any disease is caused by alteration of normal neural function — normal neural function can be altered as a result of misalignments of the spinal vertebrae (subluxations). These subluxations disturb the spinal nerves in their mediation of mind and body and inhibit the vital force in its attempt to maintain health.

4 'One cause, one cure' — since sickness and disease are a result of disturbed neural function, and subluxated vertebrae are the major cause of such disturbance, then elimination of spinal subluxations via chiropractic manipulation will restore health by restoring neural function and promoting the body's capacity for self-healing.

These principles are not too dissimilar to osteopathic principles. Both chiropractic and osteopathy share the view that the body's various 'parts' (i.e. organs, tissues, cells) are interrelated and that health is dependent on this relationship. They both recognise the interdependence of structure and function, and both approaches acknowledge the importance of the body's self-healing capacity (i.e. vital force) in maintaining and restoring health.

Chiropractic manipulative techniques

Most chiropractors today restrict their manipulations to the spinal column and pelvis. Some chiropractors perform adjustments to the bones of the skull. Some also manipulate or adjust the joints of the body's extremities. Chiropractic manipulative technique consists mainly of high velocity, low amplitude (HVLA) thrusting adjustments. The aim of these adjustments is to increase mobility of the spinal joints and eliminate spasms in the associated muscles, thereby enabling the spinal nerves to function effectively. Box 1.2 outlines the most commonly used chiropractic techniques. However, it should be noted that members of the profession use numerous other adjustment techniques.

A chiropractic consultation and treatment involves the taking of a thorough case history, followed by a physical examination of the spine. X-rays of the spine are often requested to assist in the formulation of a diagnosis and treatment plan; then follows the chiropractic treatment. Sometimes hot packs or massage are used to help relax muscles prior to the adjustment. Chiropractors may also recommend exercise therapy or offer lifestyle management advice to their clients (Kleynhans, Sweaney & Hunt 2003).

While in the past practitioners of chiropractic fully believed that all illness was the result of subluxation and could therefore be effectively treated with chiropractic adjustment, this view has changed. Most chiropractors today view their profession as a form of complementary therapy, which assists in the prevention and treatment of ill-health.

Physiotherapy

Physiotherapy began to develop as a profession in Australia after 1939 with the establishment of the Australian Physiotherapy Association (formerly the Australian Massage Association). From that time physiotherapy developed a strong reputation and a growing popularity in Australia and massage went into something of a decline during that period (see Chapter 2). Probably the main difference between the two professions was that physiotherapy focused more on rehabilitation from injury. This was largely due to the increased demand for rehabilitation services and skills as a result of World War II casualties.

Although massage techniques formed the foundation of physiotherapy practice, exercise therapy, thermotherapy, hydrotherapy and electrotherapy began to play an increasing part. Spinal manipulations also began to feature more frequently, especially where neck and back pain was concerned. Since that time physiotherapy has continued to develop as a profession, with government registration in all Australian states, university degree education programs and WorkCover recognition of its services. Geoff Maitland, a prominent South Australian physiotherapist, has been an influential figure in the development of manipulative physiotherapy in Australia. His techniques and approach to manipulative therapy have had a significant influence on orthopaedic manipulative therapy worldwide.

Physiotherapy's main focus is the restoration of physical function, and an understanding of the musculoskeletal system is the therapist's key area of expertise. Manipulative therapy, prescription of therapeutic exercise and electrophysical therapy (e.g. ultrasound) are used as the primary tools for minimising physical dysfunction, restoring normal function and relieving pain. While a recent trend in manipulative therapies has seen a reduction in the use of HVLA thrusting adjustments, these still form a significant part of physiotherapy. However, a greater emphasis on rehabilitative exercise therapy is evident in most physiotherapy practices.

These days, physiotherapy training incorporates such specialty areas as neurological, cardiothoracic, paediatric, gerontological and of course, musculoskeletal physiotherapy. With health assessment there is now greater emphasis on identifying the dysfunction, its source and also the causes of the source of dysfunction, and factors contributing to it, rather than simply determining the pathophysiology. Health evaluation has become more client-centred, and the bio-psychological perspective of the dysfunction has overshadowed a patho-biological

---

Box 1.2 Chiropractic treatment techniques

- Receptor-tonus method (Nimmo technique) — improves muscle function and postural balance via techniques that eliminate trigger points.
- Diversified — delivered to individual or groups of vertebral segments.
- Gonstead — direct thrust in the direction opposite to that of the motion restriction (i.e. similar to osteopathic indirect technique).
- Activator — use of a spring-loaded gun-like device to deliver very high velocity force to vertebrae and sometimes soft tissues such as muscles or ligaments.
- Thompson Terminal Point — HVLA adjustment to the spine, especially the pelvis, using a specialised treatment table.
- Logan basic — fascial release technique to the sacrotuberous ligament for the purpose of correcting subluxation of the sacrum.
- Flexion distraction — traction-mobilisation for treatment of intervertebral disc problems.
- Hole-in-one technique — focuses on manipulation of the first two cervical vertebrae since these were seen to be crucial to the alignment of all other spinal vertebrae.
- Sacro-occipital technique — aims to achieve balance and alignment between the pelvis and the spine, thus enhancing the flow of cerebro-spinal fluid to optimise nerve function.
- Applied kinesiology — based on the concept that vertebral subluxations create specific muscle weaknesses; used to diagnose vertebral misalignment and to correct associated muscle weakness.

understanding. Patho-biological diagnosis serves mainly to identify precautions and contraindications to the treatment and management of the problem (Maitland 2001). Clients are encouraged to participate in the process of rehabilitation as much as possible (by complying with the prescribed exercise regime).

Physiotherapy manipulative techniques

Manipulative physiotherapy techniques may be broadly categorised into two types, gentle pain-modulating methods and stronger mobilising techniques. The stronger mobilising techniques are similar to the HVLA methods used by chiropractors and osteopaths. They force a movement beyond its limited range of motion via a sudden thrust. The gentler methods coax a movement by passive rhythmical oscillations performed within or at the limit of the range of motion. Most areas of the body's skeleton may be treated (i.e. not just the spine). Wherever possible the gentler methods are preferred because the client has greater control, being able to resist the mobilisation if they experience too much pain, whereas the sudden HVLA manipulation prohibits any control by the client. Manipulation of the body's soft tissues also takes place where appropriate. Massage technique is rarely used these days by physiotherapists, although techniques such as trigger-point therapy, myofascial release and muscle energy technique are being used increasingly by some therapists. Physiotherapists stress that the manipulative techniques they employ are based on scientific knowledge and research. They have not been determined empirically.

A typical physiotherapy session begins with a detailed assessment that will incorporate the taking of a case history and extensive physical examination. As previously mentioned, a client-centred approach to assessment has evolved. The physiotherapist is particularly interested in the client's expression of their signs and symptoms, and how their specific dysfunction limits and affects their activities. Diagnosis of the pathology is not the 'be all and end all'. In many cases of musculoskeletal dysfunction the pathology will not be known for certain and therefore the treatment strategy will be determined largely from the information provided by the client and the signs and symptoms he/she is presenting. Evaluation of the client's full range of motion, gait, posture and strength is usually undertaken. X-rays and CT scans may assist the therapist in determining the most appropriate treatment strategy. The treatment plan will inevitably involve stretching and exercise prescription, perhaps ultrasound or other electrophysical application, thermotherapy, and possibly manipulative therapy. Some physiotherapists include musculoskeletal acupuncture (needling or laser) to the trigger points of affected areas.

Remedial massage therapy

Manipulation of the musculoskeletal system of the body is an integral part of remedial massage. While this manipulation applies mainly to the body's soft tissues, mobilisation of joints can be part of the scope of practice of the massage therapist where adequate training in the appropriate techniques has been undertaken, and where state/territory law permits (see Chapter 5).

Remedial massage generally does not incorporate HVLA manipulations of the spine, however vertebral subluxations may be addressed by applying massage and other soft tissue techniques (for example, trigger-point therapy, post-isometric relaxation technique) to the soft tissues that support and surround the spine. Once these muscles or ligaments have been satisfactorily relaxed or returned to a balanced state, stretching and/or gentle mobilisation of the affected joints may correct the alignment of the vertebrae.

MASSAGE TRAINING

In the past, massage therapy training was largely unregulated. Prior to the mid-1990s standards and qualifications varied enormously and control of the quality of training was loose. However, national standards for the training of massage therapists were first endorsed and introduced in Australia in 2000, and reviewed in 2006. In the Vocational Education and Training (VET) sector, such standards are defined in the Health Training Package for Complementary and Alternative Therapies; which is a document that details the required skills and knowledge for the following bodywork qualifications:

- Certificate IV in Massage Therapy Practice
- Diploma of Shiatsu
- Diploma of Traditional Chinese Remedial Massage (an mo tui na)
- Diploma of Remedial Massage.

This training package aims to ensure that all Australian massage professionals in the industry at least have a minimum and consistent standard of training. This should contribute to a more consistent standard of service for Australian consumers of bodywork therapy, an increased acceptance of massage and the other bodywork methods as effective health care modalities, and an even greater confidence in natural medicine generally.

CONCLUSION

As massage therapy continues to evolve as a profession and also as a therapy, it seems likely that training programs in massage, especially remedial massage, will incorporate more advanced assessment methods and techniques of manipulation (both of soft tissues and bony structures). When this occurs, massage as a healing method will have come full circle, in that the bodywork therapists from past civilisations and from other systems of medicine always integrated the art of bonesetting with the gentle skills of soft tissue massage, corrective exercise and posture technique.

Questions and activities

1   You are designing a promotional flyer for use in your clinic.
    (a) Write a definition of massage for inclusion that makes reference to some of the original meanings of the word.

(b) Write a paragraph that outlines the major principles underpinning the practice of natural medicine.

2 A client has asked you for a referral for their gastric reflux. They are not sure whether to visit a traditional Chinese medicine (TCM) practitioner, ayurvedic practitioner or a naturopath. Describe what you would tell them in relation to these different modalities, including any aspects of their practice that are common.

3 A client asks you what the difference is between herbal medicine, homoeopathy and nutrition therapy. What would you say?

4 Prepare a statement that could be provided to clients that describes and outlines the benefits of each of the following modalities:
   (a) osteopathy
   (b) chiropractic
   (c) physiotherapy
   (d) remedial massage therapy.

Recommended reading

Grossinger R 1995 *Planet Medicine: Modalities* (6th edn). North Atlantic Books, New York

Maury M 2004 *Marguerite Maury's Guide to Aromatherapy: the Secret of Life and Youth*. Random House, UK

Micozzi MS (ed.) 2001 *Fundamentals of Complementary and Alternative Medicine*. Churchill Livingstone, New York

Novey DW 2000 *Clinician's Complete Reference to Complementary and Alternative Medicine*. Mosby, St Louis

Robson T (ed.) 2004 *An Introduction to Complementary Medicine*. Allen & Unwin, Sydney

Ward RC (ed.) 2003 *Foundations for Osteopathic Medicine* (2nd edn). Lippincott Williams & Wilkins, Philadelphia

References

Chaitow L 1996 *Muscle Energy Techniques*. Churchill Livingstone, Edinburgh

Chopra D 1987 *Creating Health*. Houghton Mifflin, Boston

—— 1989 *Quantum Healing*. Bantam Books, New York

—— 1990 *Perfect Health*. Harmony Books, New York

Collins Concise Dictionary 1989 Australian edition. Collins, London

Dvorak J, Dvorak V, Schneider W (eds) 1985 *Manual Medicine 1984*. Springer-Verlag, Heidelberg, Germany

Gallagher RM, Humphrey FJ 2001 *Osteopathic Medicine: A Reformation in Progress*. Churchill Livingstone, Philadelphia

Greenman PE 1996 *Principles of Manual Medicine*. Lippincott Williams & Wilkins, Philadelphia

House of Lords — Science and Technology — Sixth Report 2000 *Complementary and Alternative Medicine*. UK Parliament

Kaptchuk T, Croucher M 1986 *The Healing Arts: A Journey Through the Faces of Medicine*. British Broadcasting Corporation, London

Kleynhans AM, Sweaney JD, Hunt RG 2003 Chiropractic. In: Freckelton I, Selby H (eds) *Expert Evidence*. Thomson Lawbook Co. Section 4-901–1083

Maitland GD 2001 *Maitland's Vertebral Manipulation* (6th edn). Butterworth–Heinemann, Oxford

—— 2005 *Maitland's Vertebral Manipulation* (7th edn). Butterworth–Heinemann, Oxford

Maury M 2004 *Marguerite Maury's Guide to Aromatherapy: the Secret of Life and Youth*. Random House, UK

New England Journal of Medicine 1992; 326:61

Pfizer Australia Health Report 2006 *Australians and Their Medicines*. Pfizer Australia, issue 24

Pizzorno JE, Murray MT 1999 *Textbook of Natural Medicine* (2nd edn). Churchill Livingstone, London

Segen JC 1998 *Dictionary of Alternative Medicine*. Appleton & Lange, Stamford, Connecticut

Siahpush M 1998 Postmodern values, dissatisfaction with conventional medicine and popularity of alternative therapies. *Journal of Sociology*, 34(1)

Tappan F 1988 *Healing Massage Techniques: Holistic, Classic and Emerging Methods* (2nd edn). Appleton & Lange, Norwalk

Turchaninov R 2001 *Therapeutic Massage: A Scientific Approach*. Aesculapius Books, Phoenix, Arizona

World Health Organization (WHO) 1998 *Traditional Medicine*. WHO Publications, Geneva, Switzerland

a history of massage
Katharine Callaway and Susan Burgess

chapter **2**

LEARNING OUTCOMES
- Summarise the origins and history of massage
- Identify how historical events have led to current philosophies
- Develop an understanding of the importance of historical factors in the theory and practice of massage today

---

INTRODUCTION

The oldest written reference to what is now called massage is thousands of years old. As such, today's practitioners are quite possibly using skills that have been developed and refined over some 5000 years.

Knowledge of the history of massage will assist students to recognise their place in the profession and in forming their own beliefs and philosophies about how massage fits into society.

This chapter will discuss the development and growth of massage from its most primitive days to modern times. From its starting point in ancient history, this chapter moves through the 'Dark Ages' to modern times and includes contributions that early massage therapists made to the profession in Australia.

ANCIENT TIMES (3000 BC–AD 400)

There is evidence that massage was widely used in ancient times. The first recorded evidence dates back to around 2350 BC in Babylon (today's Iraq) where cuneiform text inscribed on clay tablets implied that massage was used.

Historians generally believe that Egyptian and Chinese cultures developed at around the same time; however, dating of early Chinese texts is complicated because of the tendency at the time for Chinese writers to credit their work to a previous emperor as an expression of honour.

In Egypt, foot and hand massage was documented as a form of treatment. This is evidenced by a wall painting (c. 2330 BC) in the tomb of Ankhmahor depicting a physician massaging the hands and feet of a patient. The wall painting suggests that techniques used in this form of massage were thumb and finger pressures, as well as squeezing and pressing with the fingertips. Today such techniques might be referred to as reflexology, which is a form of pressure point massage applied to the hands, feet and ears.

The Jews gained knowledge of using aromatic oils from the Egyptian embalming process, and developed anointing and rubbing rituals to cleanse and purify the body and mind.

Archaeological discoveries in China have contributed to our knowledge of the origins of massage. A text written by Unschuld (2000) makes reference to an archaeological site that discovered a funerary complex from 168 BC known as Mawangdui, near the city of Changsha in the central Chinese province of Hunan. This site uncovered 14 medical manuscripts that document medical developments during the end of the Zhou Dynasty (1122–221 BC), during the Qin dynasty (221–207 BC) and at the beginning of the Han dynasty (206–220 AD). These manuscripts, believed to constitute the oldest medical text written in China, mention many methods of healing including what is now called massage.

Another ancient text is *The Yellow Emperor's Classic of Internal Medicine* (Nei Ching). Claimed by some to be written around 2500 BC, it was more probably written around 200 BC or even later. The translation (Veith 1972) shows that massage was considered one of the five treatments of that era. It describes the treatment of paralysis, chills and fever and states that 'these diseases are most fittingly treated with breathing exercises, massage of the skin and flesh, and exercises of the hands and feet' (p 168).

In ancient times, the Chinese referred to their system of massage as *amma*, which involved techniques such as rubbing and finger pressure along the meridians of the body. These ancient hand techniques are still employed, along with additional techniques such as pulling of limbs and pushing of the soft tissues. Today's Chinese system of massage is referred to as *an mo tui na*, or traditional Chinese medicine (TCM) remedial massage.

The trade routes are believed to have resulted in a spread of massage techniques to India where it is surmised that massage was integrated with yoga to form a system of exercise and massage to promote and maintain health, spirituality and vitality. During 1800 BC, four 'books of wisdom' were written in India, based on sacred Hindu teachings known as the Vedas. Many authors believe that massage was written about in the Ayur-Veda volume. Kleen (1918: 1) states that '… Professor Pagel of Berlin [could not find] anything on these subjects in the Ayur-Veda'. Later on however, in 300 BC, the *Laws of Man* mentioned massage as a duty of everyday life. Techniques such as kneading, tapôtement, frictions and cracking are listed (Beck 1999: 6).

In Japan, the Chinese *amma* philosophy of working with the body's meridians led to the development of shiatsu therapy in the seventeenth century. This therapy, which is popular today in both Eastern and Western countries, uses thumb and finger pressure on *tsubo* points (energy points along the meridians) as the fundamental technique.

Meanwhile in Ancient Greece Asclepius (Asclepiades), a practitioner of medicine, became regarded as a god due to his healing arts. Kellogg (1895) writes:

> Asclepiades … held the practice of this art in such esteem that he abandoned the use of medicines of all sorts, relying exclusively upon massage, which he claimed effects a cure by restoring to the nutritive fluids their natural, free movements. It was this physician who made the discovery that sleep may be induced by gentle stroking.

Another legacy from Asclepius is the symbol of the medical staff with two serpents twisting around it, *cadeucus*, which is widely recognised as a symbol of medical and pharmaceutical practices.

Hippocrates of Cos (c. 460–377 BC) was a follower of Asclepius' work and was taught by Herodicus, the founder of medical gymnastics, exercise therapy for the development of the body, and for prevention and treatment of disease. Hippocrates became so famous he was given the title 'father of medicine'. He believed that medicine should be practised as an art inspired by the love of man. He chose surgery only as a last resort and preferred to use natural medicines and hands-on techniques as a primary cure or preventative. Hippocrates referred to his hands-on methods as *anatripsis* (rub). One of his most famous quotes relating to massage is (Beard & Wood 1964: 3):

> … the physician must be acquainted with many things and assuredly with anatripsis [rubbing], for things that have the same name have not the same effects. For rubbing can bind a joint that is too loose or loosen a joint that is too hard.

The conquests of Alexander the Great took the Greeks east across Asia Minor and as far as India where they learnt ayurveda, the ancient Indian system of medicine. After their return to the Mediterranean in 327 BC, soldiers are reported to have used the Indian art of head massage known as champissage.

Many Greek physicians began arriving in Rome. They were originally treated as slaves, but their medical expertise was gradually recognised and they were granted the rights of free citizens. Their treatment methods, including massage, were spread throughout the entire empire across Europe reaching as far north as Britain. Julius Caesar and Pliny the Elder are both said to have endorsed and received regular massage treatments.

Originally from Greece, Claudius Galen (AD 130–199) followed Hippocrates' work and became a prominent physician of this time. As physician to the gladiators he used massage techniques to treat injuries. Galen's experience with the gladiators confirmed his belief in the validity of massage as a treatment. In Rome he lectured and gave physical demonstrations on the theory and practice of medicine. He also wrote over 400 books on medical practices, including massage and gymnastics (Chandler 1980).

At much the same time in Rome, the physician Aulus Celsus (AD 129–199) published his *De Medicina*, in which rubbing and exercises are strongly favoured as a form of therapeutic relief.

Bathing culture in Greece and Rome

The bathing culture, as used by the Greeks and Romans, highlights one way in which massage was employed during ancient times. Around 400 BC large gymnasiums (known as *esclapeion*) were built close to town or by the seashore and they were dedicated to healing, education and public discourse. In the centre of these palatial gymnasiums was the young men's hall where athletes and citizens discussed the tactics of sport and politics and would rest and massage each other (Calvert, 2002).

The Roman baths were as important as the Greek gymnasiums and followed similar themes. By the last century BC, they 'took on an importance unparalleled in human history' (Calvert 2002). The following is a testimony to the value the Romans placed on massage (cited in Calvert 2002: 60):

> The wise and able Emperor Hadrian, 76–138 AD, who will be so well remembered as having built the wall from the Solway Firth to the Tyne, and whose reign was distinguished by peace and beneficent energy, one day saw a veteran soldier rubbing himself against the marble at the public baths, and asked him why he did so. The veteran answered, 'I have no slave to rub me,' where upon the emperor gave him two slaves and gold sufficient to maintain them. Another day several old men rubbed themselves against the wall in the emperor's presence, hoping for similar good fortune, when the shrewd Hadrian, perceiving their object, directed them to rub one another!

THE DARK AGES/MIDDLE AGES (AD 400–1450)

The early Middle Ages are often referred to as the Dark Ages because of the low level of learning or 'enlightenment'. During this time information was lost, new

2 A history of massage   13

material was not written and, in most of Europe, Christianity had a huge hold over the beliefs of men and women.

By the end of the fifth century the Roman Empire was overrun by warring tribes. As a result of such invasions, works like *De Medicina* that Celsus wrote were 'lost'. Christianity gradually became a permeating influence and knowledge was closely guarded and moderated by the monks, who were the Christian scholars of the time. Anything that was considered to be heretical or non-Christian was not released to the Christian people. Christians did use touching as a part of their beliefs and it was referred to as the 'laying on of hands', however the use of the body for pleasure was discouraged and seen as sinful. Folk healers may have been the only people who practised massage during this time, but due to the beliefs about sinful behaviour being against Christian doctrine, they were dubbed as going against God's will and were often punished for their actions.

While Christianity was being established in the West, a new religion and way of life, which is now known as Islam, was founded in Arabia by the prophet Mohammad (c. 570–632). Around AD 750 the art of making paper reached the Islamic world from China, thus allowing new and rediscovered works to be transcribed. In time this learning reached Western Europe via Spain, where Islam had become established.

As a result of this, the lost work of Hippocrates, Galen and Celsus was revived and spread throughout Europe.

During the ninth and tenth centuries new medical texts were written. Some of the work of the Islamic–Persian philosopher/physician Rhazes, or Razi, (860–932) was based on the work of Hippocrates and Galen. Razi wrote an encyclopaedia in which he praised and promoted massage, as well as exercise and diet, to maintain health and wellbeing. Another great Persian philosopher/physician, Avicenna (980–1037) wrote the *Canon of Medicine*, basing his beliefs about medicine on Galen's work and promoting the use of massage and exercise.

In about 1450 Johannes Gutenberg and his colleagues brought together the elements of modern printing for the first time. It was this creation of the Gutenberg press that allowed works such as *De Medicina* by Celsus to be circulated through the greater world once again.

THE MODERN ERA (1450–2000)

About 100 years later, well into the Renaissance, French physician Ambrois Paré (c. 1510–1590) wrote about the use of massage as a treatment. Paré was mainly interested in the effects of massage on broken joints or after orthopaedic surgery. He referred to the speeds and depths with which frictions were applied to the body, plus mobilisation of the joints (Palmer 1912). Today these techniques are constantly employed by massage therapists.

In 1569, Girolamo Mercuriale (1530–1606) wrote *De Arte Gymnastica*, following the theme that massage and exercise were a partnership to be used during the same session.

Records show that a physician named Hoffman (1660–1742) used massage and exercise as part of his medical practice in Germany. Along with exercise, he used massage in the way that Hippocrates, Galen and Celsus advocated. Hoffman's work contributed to the medical practices in Germany, France and England and paved the way for the public to become aware of the benefits of massage and exercise.

Per Henrik Ling (1776–1839) was born in Sweden and, with two French associates, set the wheels in motion to produce *Svenska Gymnastikens* (Swedish Exercise), which today is known as Swedish massage. In 1804 Ling began lecturing at the Lunds Universitet on the art of fencing and gymnastics. He studied anatomy and physiology and further developed his knowledge of how the human body moves. While teaching fencing to his students, Ling noted that some students could not physically perform the moves he wanted them to. He learnt through teaching gymnastics to his students that posture could be re-educated to produce greater efficiency of movement.

Ling opened the Swedish Royal Central Institute of Gymnastics in 1813, where he continued the development of his ideas. Salvo (1999: 10) quotes Ling as saying: '[we] try by means of influencing movements to alleviate or overcome sufferings that have arisen through abnormal conditions'. Ling began to classify his gymnastic movements into *active* (performed by the client alone), *passive* (movements of the client's limbs performed by the therapist) and *duplicated* (performed by the client with assistance from the therapist). Ling's 'passive movement' incorporated massage techniques such as friction, hacking, pinching, squeezing and kneading.

By 1851, Ling's teachings had spread to 38 schools throughout Europe. However, Ling's name was exploited to market Swedish gymnastics and this brought his developments to the attention of the medical fraternity, who ridiculed his work on the basis that his education in anatomy and physiology was not extensive. Despite this, Ling's work did receive a favourable reception in parts of Europe.

In Holland, Dr Johann Mezger (1839–1909) and an English physician, Mathias Roth, have been credited for bringing Ling's work to the scientific community. Mezger introduced the terminology still used today, such as effleurage, pétrissage, tapôtement (including beating and clapping) and massage (Beard & Wood 1964). Mezger spread massage into Germany and Austria, through his extensive practice of this art and his ability to competently display its benefits to others in the medical profession.

The French physician Just Marie Marcellin Lucas-Championnière claimed, in about 1880, that 'in fractures, the soft tissue union as well as the bony union should be considered from the start' (Tappan 1988: 7). Lucas-Championnière's ideas impressed Sir William Bennett who began using massage to treat patients at St Georges Hospital in England during the late nineteenth century. The validation of massage by Bennett and Roth influenced British opinion as to its worth. Mennell later writes 'those who have once seen the treatment first devised by Lucas-Championnière applied to a recent fracture cannot but admit that they have witnessed the result of a profound reflex' (1920: 6).

Interest in massage was not limited to Europe. In the US in 1856, two brothers, Charles and George Taylor, introduced Ling's work. They learned the techniques from Roth and were the driving force behind Americans' belief in the benefits of massage. By 1880, medical research had begun in New York on the benefits of massage in the management of anaemia.

Back in London, specifically during 1894, the British Medical Association (BMA) made a special inquiry into the education and practice of massage practitioners. This inquiry, which fuelled the 'Massage Scandals of 1894', found that many schools of massage were using questionable tactics to enrol students. Graduates of these schools were usually unskilled and in debt and were offered employment by their schools. However, it was not unknown for this employment to include prostitution. Thus the longstanding association between massage and prostitution was reinforced. The term 'massage parlour' as a euphemism for brothels was popularised by this scandal. In addition, the BMA's inquiry found that qualifications had been forged, leading to public mistrust.

A group of women started the first massage association in London, named the Society of Trained Masseuses. They hoped to gain acceptance of massage as a legitimate field of study and an emerging career option and profession. The women used the medical model to shape their society, making high academic standards a part of the compulsory entrance requirements. Training was only done at selected schools, and these schools were monitored regularly to maintain the society's standards.

Over the next hundred years, many types of massage and bodywork developed. In 1920 Dr James Mennell divided massage effects into two categories — mechanical actions and reflex actions. Mennell showed that massaging a patient produced mechanical actions such as moving venous blood and lymph, and also stretched connective tissue affecting tendons and scar tissue. Mennell noted that when stimulating the tactile skin receptors, reflex action occurring to soft tissue such as muscle caused it to relax or contract, depending on the type of stroke used.

About 15 years later a Danish physiologist, Emil Vodder, along with his wife Estris, developed *manual lymphatic drainage*, which uses very light circular motion on the skin to work directly with the lymphatic system. In 1936 the Vodders' presented their work to a congress in Paris. Whilst in France, Emil Vodder was working as a medical massage therapist on English clients with chronic sinusitis, acne and migraine. He noted these patients had swollen lymph glands in the cervical region. It was taboo in medical profession of this time to stimulate the lymphatic systems for fear of spreading disease but Vodder and his wife discovered the swelling could be relieved by using light, pumping, circular movements in the direction of the lymph flow.

However it was not until the 1960s, after Dr Asdonk from Germany had conducted research on 20 000 patients using the Vodder method, that manual lymphatic drainage became accepted in conventional medical institutions. Dr Vodder passed on his life work to

his colleagues, Guenther and Hildegard Wittlinger from Austria. The Wittlingers established the Dr Vodder School in 1971 where the family continue Dr Vodder's work and teach his method in its original form, which is considered to represent the gold standard in manual lymphatic drainage today. The work has spread worldwide and a number of practitioners in Australia are specially trained in this technique today.

> Vodder always saw the human as a whole. His thesis was 'if one part is sick the whole human being is sick'. He only gave whole body treatments with special dedication to the affected area.
>
> *(Wittlinger 2004)*

Soft tissue manipulations were also popularised at this time. In Germany Elizabeth Dick developed *bindgewebs* (connective tissue) massage in 1929. In England an orthopaedic surgeon, James Cyriax, developed *transverse friction massage*. Cyriax set up a department at St Thomas's hospital in London, in 1938. It was dedicated to developing massage and manipulation, and later became the department of orthopaedic medicine. He is credited today as the father of orthopaedic medicine. Cyriax published the *Textbook of Orthopedic Medicine: Volume 2* (11th edn, 1984), and this laid the foundation for soft tissue manipulations.

Massage in Europe — World War I to the present

Throughout the two world wars, massage was frequently used to help the rehabilitation of service men in the Allied forces hospitals. Inside Nazi territory Felix Kersten (1898–1960), a manual therapist trained in Sweden, was obligated to use massage and pressure point techniques to relieve Reichfuhrer SS Himmler of his severe stomach pains. Before the war, Kersten had worked in Finland, Sweden and Holland. He was apparently so effective in treating Himmler that he was able to use his position to help many people escape the death camps (Calvert 2002). From 1945 massage was being performed in athletic clubs and YMCAs for the benefit of athletes and sportsmen.

The popularity of massage grew in Europe in the 1960s and became a more commonly utilised form of therapy in the 1970s. Increased interest in alternative therapies opened up opportunities to explore different techniques of bodywork which came to Europe from America and Asia. Narendra Mehta introduced *Indian head massage* to London in 1981 at the Mind, Body, Spirit exhibition in Olympia. Mehta integrated classic massage with Indian head massage and traditional Indian Ayurvedic techniques to successfully create a treatment that combined both eastern and western massage methods. In the 1990s he went on to develop a qualification in Indian head massage that is now recognised internationally (Mehta 2000).

More recently Mary D Nelson from Tucson, America has bought to Europe her version of hot stone massage. In 1993, Nelson discovered how the benefits of using hot and cold balsam stones helped enhance the effects of a wide variety of massage techniques. She built upon and experimented with the different ways the stones could be used on the body using modern and ancient traditions from Asia and native American Indians. Today, her workshops have become popular amongst therapy schools within Europe and worldwide.

The growth of massage and complementary therapies in the UK has increased as has the requirement for professional regulation. The Federation of Holistic Therapists (FHT) was established in 1962 to represent and support multi-disciplinary therapists, promoting high standards in education, regulation and professional practices for sports, beauty and complementary therapy. Complementary therapies growth in the UK also led the National Health Service (NHS) to set up a directory of complementary and alternative practitioners. In 1993, HRH Prince Charles founded The Princes Foundation of Integrated Health to promote a holistic approach to medical care in the UK. Initially only modalities such as osteopathy and chiropractic were registered. But, on 31 March 2008 a reception was held in the presence of the British Minister of State for Health Services to celebrate the formation of the Complementary and Natural Healthcare Council. This council has been set up to regulate massage and other complementary therapists within the UK.

> We are infinitely complex beings — mind, body and spirit — that cannot just be reduced to mechanical functioning. Healthcare should, and must, attend appropriately to all three aspects
>
> *(HRH The Prince of Wales 2008)*

MASSAGE IN AUSTRALIA
The Aboriginal connection

The healing methods used by the early Aboriginal people were, and still are, based on mind, body, spirit, socio-community, and environment. Approaches to healing among the Aborigines appear to vary according to region. When interviewed on 4 March 2003 Ann Warren, an Aboriginal elder from the Dtjilmamidtung region, states that 'the healings that take place cannot be compartmentalised into any one modality'. What this means is that the Aborigines do not recognise the word massage, however they do recognise the practice of touch. Warren also describes the healings as 'wholistic', whereby every part of the being is considered and the person is treated as a whole. Warren describes a method of using touch as a healing instrument in the Dtjilmamidtung region as follows (2003):

> You may have a group of women in a circle exchanging words and sharing experiences. In this group there would be children sitting across laps or lying in between two people. Everyone who makes the circle would be touching in some way. Their knees may be touching the person on either side of them or they may be holding hands. As the exchange and sharing progresses, one woman may get a feeling about another woman that something is up for her. This woman would then rub, touch and soothe the other woman

with a great respect for personal boundaries, and the energy of the group, and would then ask if everything was OK. This in itself is how a healing may take place. The intention of the touch is to project healing rather than to specifically manipulate the body's soft tissue. The touch and concern of the first woman transfers into the second woman and the whole circle would be affected by this movement, the children would also be affected and then they learn how to intuit that something is up for someone, usually for their mothers and use this touch to transmit healing energy.

The period 1870–1920

By the 1870s massage therapists were known to be practising in Melbourne and Sydney. There were different ways of obtaining a massage, including referral to private rooms by medical practitioners where massage was performed by therapists who had gained credible reputations.

According to Dunstan and Bentley (2000), in 1880 an Australian doctor, Louis Henry, placed massage as 'a third branch of medical practice on equal footing with surgery and medicine'. This statement helped to pave the way for massage to be accepted as a mainstream therapy. Practitioners such as Teepoo Hall (1860–1909) became well regarded as massage therapists. Hall worked with the surgeon Thomas Fitzgerald (1838–1908) and his clients included several dignitaries. He practised at what is now the Austin and Repatriation Medical Centre (Austin Hospital) and became one of the first clinical teachers of massage, rising to the position of senior masseur and demonstrator at the Melbourne Hospital.

Likewise, Alfred Peters (1871–1944), who emigrated to Australia from England, started working as a masseur in Melbourne hospitals. He treated many sportsmen and also the Russian ballerina, Anna Pavlova. When Peters emigrated to Australia he advocated the benefits of massage and the medical profession could not ignore his claims. In his book, *Massage: Its History, Its Curative Uses and Its Practical Results* (1890), Peters refers to massage as 'one of the simplest, most rational, most efficacious and most valuable of curative agencies' (p 3).

Figure 2.1 depicts massage in Australia before 1905.

Around 1912 a masseur by the name of Joseph Fay wrote a text titled *Scientific Massage for Athletes*. The title page heralded him as 'The Australian Authority On Massage For Athletes' and this text may well have been the first sports massage text written in Australia. Fay described what distinguishes an average massage therapist from a practical massage therapist, namely 'the former one merely pats or plays with the hide [skin], while the latter works with the meat, or muscle, between the hide and the bone so that it is in its highest state for exercise'. Fay classified three main massage movements as friction, kneading and vibration. In his text he described a method to massage the whole body such that it is done in a systemic and organised fashion (Fay c. 1912).

By 1905, massage societies were in existence in New South Wales, Victoria and South Australia. In 1906 a meeting chaired by Dr John Springthorpe resulted in the formation of the national Australasian Massage

By 1905, massage societies were in existence in New South Wales, Victoria and South Australia. In 1906 a meeting chaired by Dr John Springthorpe resulted in the formation of the national Australasian Massage Association (AMA) and Peters was an integral influence in this association. By 25 April 1907 membership totals for the AMA stood at 302: New South Wales 112; Victoria 141; South Australia 15; Queensland 12; Western Australia 3; Tasmania 12 and New Zealand 7. Also there was a total of 196 honorary medical members on the books. Although today each state has its own massage association, a comparison has been made to indicate the membership growth of the professional massage associations: New South Wales 1200; Victoria and Tasmania 1616; South Australia and Northern Territory 650; Queensland 1100; Western Australia 200; and New Zealand 460.

Figure 2.1 Massage in Australia before 1905

Association (AMA) and Peters was an integral influence in this association. By 25 April 1907 membership totals for the AMA stood at 302: New South Wales 112; Victoria 141; South Australia 15; Queensland 12; Western Australia 3; Tasmania 12 and New Zealand 7. Also there were a total of 196 honorary medical members on the books. Although today each state has its own massage association, a comparison has been made to indicate the membership growth of the professional massage associations: New South Wales 1200; Victoria and Tasmania 1616; South Australia and Northern Territory 650; Queensland 1100; Western Australia 200; and New Zealand 460.

Australia at war

When World War I began, members of the AMA made applications to serve as massage therapists, but were turned down by the Australian Imperial Forces. Their spirit remained steady and strong and as Butler (1943: 595) states '… the practitioners of massage were enthusiastic and, there can be no doubt, convinced believers in the value of their art and of the importance of its proper application'.

After several further unsuccessful attempts, approval was finally given in 1915, due largely to the constant pressure from the AMA. As recorded by Butler (1943: 597):

> The dispatch of a party or section of masseurs in the proportion of 1 male to 2 females, males to have pay and privileges of staff-sergeants, females pay and privileges of staff nurses. Under these conditions they must be prepared to serve for the term of war, and wear a uniform as directed for which allowance will be made.

One staff member alone would treat 15 cases a day. A report made by Colonel McWhae to General Howse states the following (Butler 1943: 613):

> All soldiers with stiffness of joints, contractures of muscles or tendons and similar lesions will receive remedial gymnastic treatment, providing no acute inflammation, oedema or unhealed wounds (except in special selected cases of the latter) are present. e.g. Stiffness of the shoulder, elbow or wrist, limitation of extension of the elbow, limitation of supination and pronation of the forearm, stiffness of the wrist, hand or fingers with contractures and loss of handgrip, stiffness of the knee whether accompanied or not by a flexion, contracture, stiffness or limited mobility of

the ankle, contracture of the calf muscle with resultant foot drop deformities of the foot, etc.

The AMA fought a huge battle of its own during WWI, striving for recognition. Eventually its efforts were noticed but ironically they underwent the same challenges in WWII. Butler (1943: 625) wrote:

> This much at least is certain: whatever be the future of the Australian Service of Massage, its members can be assured that their art and technique will rest now on a scientific basis of clinical and experimental research. And for this they, and medical science in general, owe a tribute to the pioneers of the war of 1914–1918.

Modern times in Australia

In 1939 the AMA changed its name to the Australian Physiotherapy Association. Massage courses became less available during the next two decades. Physiotherapy was growing in popularity and the two fields began to separate. There are different theories about why this separation occurred. One theory is that of time management. To conduct a massage can take 15 to 90 minutes, resulting in fewer patients being seen in one day, whereas a physical therapy session is quicker and more patients can be treated per day. Another theory is that the use of machines may be far less invasive for some people than to have another human touch their body.

In Melbourne in the 1960s many people were treated by Bill Mitchell, who was a trainer at the South Melbourne Football Club. No appointments were available, so patients would arrive at the clubrooms and wait in turn, then be called in and treated. Mitchell would watch a client walk towards him and by the time that client reached him he would have a fair idea of what the problem was. Payment was made by placing a donation in a tin that sat on a shelf near the exit door. Mitchell was known only through word of mouth, but his reputation was huge. One reason that Mitchell was so popular was that he treated just about every size, shape, age and type of person. He treated football players, grandmothers, adolescents and business folk, but he had a hidden talent that made him a legend in Victoria, and that was charm. Mitchell, after watching patients walk across the floor, would greet patients with a handshake, look them right in the eye and through a smiling face say 'I can fix that for yah!'. This was not always the case, but people did not seem to mind as he had more successful treatments than unsuccessful.

At the St Kilda Football Club the head trainer Jim Clancy used some of the methods that the Romans used when treating their athletes in Ancient Rome. One method Jim employed was using a strigil on the players. This device was shaped liked a spoon and could remove the dust and sweat from the players before the massage was administered.

During the early 1960s two brothers, Harry and Arthur King, from Collingwood Football Club, established a trainer's college that taught students the art of massage, training methods and assessment of player injuries. This training school is still operating from Hawthorn Football Club today.

Keith Cleaver was also in the football trade and worked for Richmond Football Club from 1955 until the 1990s. Keith learned some of his skills from Mitchell. In 1977 Cleaver became head trainer for the club. He made several suggestions to the club that a freezer be installed in the clubrooms so they could have ice on hand to treat their player's injuries. Finally, in the 1980s, the club agreed to this and that put an end to the trainers rushing out on footy morning to purchase a dozen bags of ice to have on hand for the match (confirmed by Keith Cleaver, personal communication, 17 April 2003).

Events during the 1970s were absolutely vital for the survival of massage therapy. The Esalen Institute in California was established and influenced thousands of people in America, Australia, Europe and elsewhere about awareness of body, mind and spirit. The concept of 'holism', that we are much more than just our physical body, and that each aspect is interrelated, re-emerged as an important consideration in health care. 'Alternative' health care, based on age-old, traditional healing methods from across the globe, enjoyed a revival in the West. Touch was integral to this philosophy and therefore massage fitted in with it perfectly. It could affect not only the physical aspect, but also the mind and spirit of a recipient. The Esalen Institute became a public platform for many people to introduce their work, including that of bodywork greats such as Ida Rolf and Moshe Feldenkrais. These contemporary philosophies and concepts significantly influenced the growth, development and popularity of massage therapy in Australia.

MASSAGE IN NEW ZEALAND

The approach to health and wellness adopted by Maori people is very much intertwined with their way of life. Traditionally, massage (mirimiri), herbal medicine (rongoa) and spiritual healing (wairua) formed the cornerstones of holistic Maori health care. Today, mirimiri or massage is still widely practised in Maori circles by Maori healers.

According to Riley (1994), the use of mirimiri by Maori people dates back centuries. Herbal or animal oils were often used as lubricants in the application of the three main types of massage — roromi, toto and takahi. Roromi (or romiromi), usually administered by older women, was practised daily on the adults and involved squeezing and pinching strokes, whilst toto was a form of infant massage, often used to 'correct' or alter the

infant structurally. For example, it was common practice to bend the thumb of female infants backwards so that when older, they may be better able to weave flax. It was a belief that the best person to perform takahi massage was someone who entered the world via a breach birth. Such people, born 'feet first', were thought destined to practise takahi massage, which involved walking on parts that were sore or injured to relieve muscular stiffness (Riley 1994). Such forms of massage have been passed down the generations, and are used today by many Maori health networks. Parallelling the use of this traditional form of massage was the development in the early twentieth century of modern massage practices.

The development of modern massage in New Zealand followed similar lines to that of Australia. According to Anderson (1977) there were over 300 massage therapists established in New Zealand by the early 1900s. Some of these therapists held formal massage qualifications obtained through studies overseas, whilst others had trained in New Zealand under the guidance of self-appointed massage teachers. In addition, some therapists received training in massage whilst nursing at the Auckland Hospital. Many of these massage therapists had their own practices and it was not uncommon for husbands and wives to work together.

By 1913 a massage department had been established in the Dunedin Hospital. A Mr Booth acted as Honorary Masseur within this department and later became a massage instructor to students when the department formed a school of massage. At this time an increasing number of the medical profession were becoming aware of the use and need for massage, and the importance of adequate massage training was apparent. The New Zealand branch of the British Medical Association (BMA) addressed this concern by establishing the School of Massage in Dunedin in conjunction with the Dunedin Hospital, under the auspices of the University of Otago. After administration difficulties, full responsibility of the school was transferred to the Otago Hospital Board. This board conducted examinations and issued certificates in massage, as well as medical gymnastics and the use of medical electricity (Anderson 1977).

The government of the time was aware of these activities, and considered legal registration for all practising massage therapists. This consideration was postponed due to the great war and was acted upon shortly after when the *Masseurs Registration Act* of 1920 came into force (Sanford 2003). In 1949 this Act was modified to the *Physiotherapy Act* (which is still in existence today) and massage therapy fell under the umbrella of physiotherapy. Those who wanted to practise massage and become registered had to adhere to the *Physiotherapy Act* and were required to undertake 600 hours of training.

Decades passed until, in 1985, a man by the name of Bill Wareham called all massage therapists in the Auckland area to a meeting. The intention Wareham had was to form an institute of massage therapists. This first meeting was fruitful and the Massage Institute of New Zealand Incorporated (MINZI) became an entity.

Wareham was a massage educator during this time and he would offer his students the opportunity to become members of the institute. In 1987 Wareham travelled to Wellington where he conducted some massage education and it was during his stay that the Wellington branch of MINZI was established and Auckland became head office. The MINZI (now Massage New Zealand, MNZ) has focused its efforts on the education of massage therapists and the standards of massage teachers throughout New Zealand. They have more massage teachers on the books than massage therapists but consider all types of members to be equal. MINZI supports and assists members to obtain higher education and qualifications. MINZI run annual conferences over a three-day period where massage therapists can attend a wide range of workshops to develop and maintain their skills (Tall 2003, personnel communication).

In the late 1980s a massage therapist named Jim Sandford invited fellow practitioners from around the country to a meeting to convey his perceived need for a professional body for therapeutic massage therapists. This initial meeting led some time later to the formation of the New Zealand Association of Therapeutic Massage Practitioners (NZATMP), a national professional body established to service the therapeutic massage profession in New Zealand.

Thus the newly formed association was up and running and set about addressing such concerns as education and training of therapeutic massage therapists, standards of professionalism amongst practitioners and recognition of the profession of therapeutic massage in New Zealand. NZATMP duly became an incorporated society in September 1989 and has since grown from strength to strength. Perhaps the most notable achievements of NZATMP have been in the area of developing, establishing and implementing a comprehensive program of education for individuals interested in pursuing training in therapeutic massage. Today the association has grown to include members nationwide and has recently changed its name to the Therapeutic Massage Association (TMA). The TMA's main function today is to keep a register of massage therapists who have the National Diploma of Therapeutic Massage and to foster the ongoing training, development and mentoring of massage therapists (Vautier 2003, personal communication).

FUTURE OF MASSAGE

In the UK, the House of Lords Science and Technology Committee is starting to develop ways of monitoring the use of complementary and alternative medicine (CAM). Due to the large use of CAM, issues have arisen about:

- what structures and regulations are in place with practitioners of CAM to protect the public
- whether the practitioners' level of training is adequate
- whether evidence has been accumulated and what research is being carried out
- whether there are adequate information sources on the subject

- whether the National Health Service will provide for these treatments.

At this time in order for Australian massage therapists to be considered for registration, massage would need to pose a significant health risk, and the industry would need to present a unified lobbying position. Government regulation might also follow if massage gained suitable scientific credibility, which could be achieved through conducting research programs. However, the most common way that research is achieved is when courses are at a certain academic standard. In Australia massage is, at highest, a diploma qualification. However, degrees in musculoskeletal therapy and myotherapy can now be studied and the need for research has been addressed.

The Australian Association of Massage Therapists (AAMT) has launched the Australian Massage Research Foundation (AMRF) which primarily exists to provide grants for massage related research which will contribute to the health benefits of massage.

In America massage research commenced around 1880. Since then the Institute of Touch has been developed at the Miami Medical School, where research is conducted to validate the benefits of massage. This research, sponsored by Johnson and Johnson, aims to look at the value of massage when used with infants, for postnatal depression, with premature babies and during pregnancy. In addition, text has arisen from this region of the world describing how to conduct research as a massage therapist.

CONCLUSION

An appreciation of the history of massage provides the therapist with the ability to place current knowledge into an historical and developmental context, enabling the therapist to tell people briefly about its 5000 year lineage — how it survived even through the Dark Ages, the main figures in its history and the scandals that occurred along the way. The therapist can explain the fight that massage had to undertake to serve injured men during World War I, and how beneficial the massage service was in that time.

Despite the growth of competing forms of treatment through the ages, massage has survived. Though the art of massage has sometimes faced extinction, somewhere, sometime throughout these threats, someone believed in it enough to speak highly of it and thereby influence the views of the public and medical fraternity. Current massage students represent the future of massage. In time, their work will become the history for new practitioners. As inheritors of the traditions of Hippocrates, Galen, Celsus, Avicenna, Ling, Mezger and Peters, students can think about the future of massage, what it means to them, what impact they will have on this 5000 year-old art and what direction the profession will take. Figure 2.2 is a time line of the history of massage as a healing method. It illustrates the progression and decline of massage therapy throughout history.

The arrows indicate the highs and lows of massage as a progressive healing method

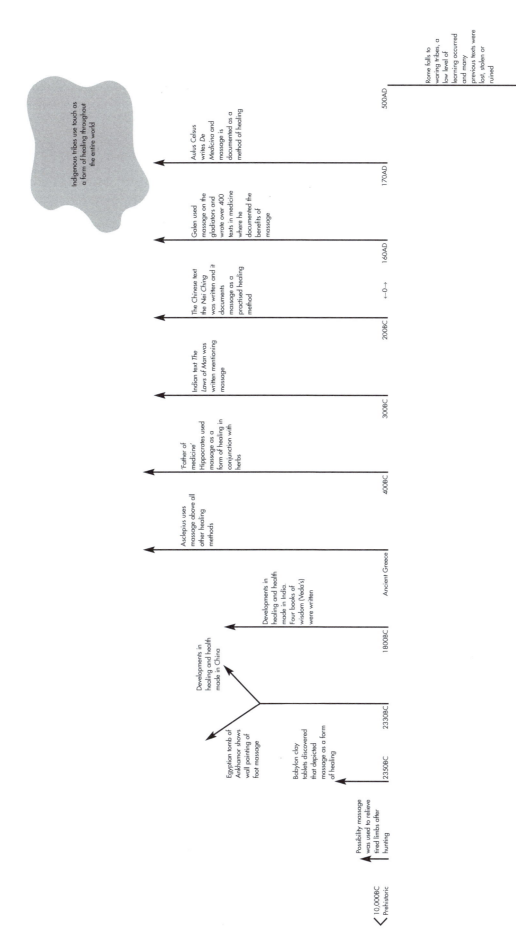

Figure 2.2 Time line of historical events

The arrows indicate the highs and lows of massage as a progressive healing method

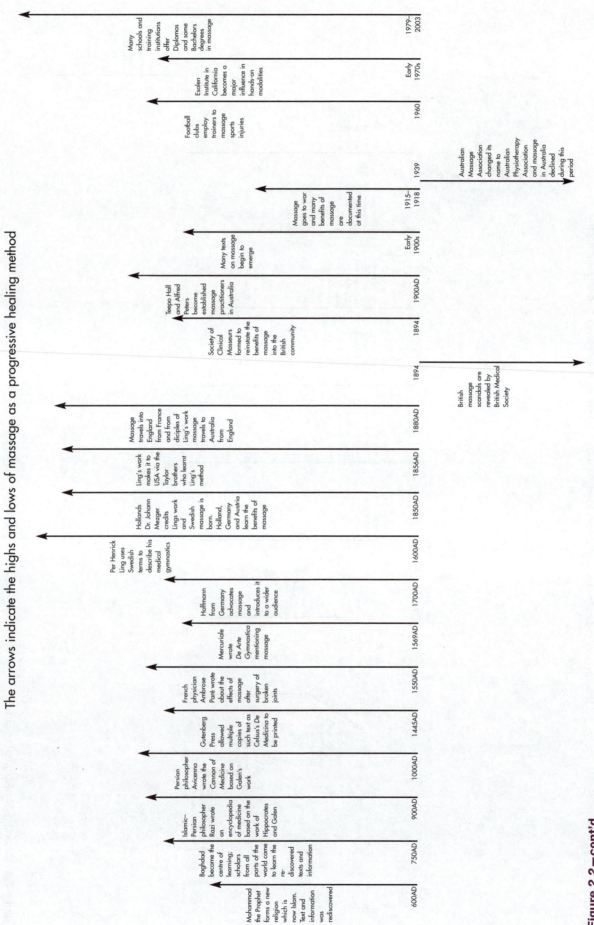

Figure 2.2—cont'd

Questions and activities

1   You have been asked to present a talk to the local Rotary group on the benefits of massage. One Rotarian inquires about the development of modern massage. Detail your response to this question, making reference to the contributions of Ling.
2   Prepare a one-page visual handout that could be used for a short presentation on massage, which illustrates a timeline of significant historical events in the development of massage therapy.
3   Describe what prompted you to be drawn to the practice of massage, and define your own personal philosophies of massage.
4   It is a fact that as recently as the eighteenth and nineteenth centuries, medical physicians used massage therapy as a form of treatment. Despite the acceptance of massage then, today massage therapists are being required to scientifically validate the use of massage as a form of therapy. Why do you think this is the case?

Recommended reading

Butler AG 1943 *The Official History of the Australian Army Medical Services in the War of 1914–1918, vol. 3*. Special Problems and Services. Australian War Memorial, Canberra

Calvert RN 2002 *The History of Massage: An Illustrated Survey From Around the World*. Healing Arts Press, Rochester

Kakkib li' Dthia Warrawee'a 2002 *There Was Once a Tree Called Deru*. HarperCollins Publishers, Sydney

Peters A 1890 *Massage: Its History, Its Curative Uses, and Its Practical Results*. Public Library, Melbourne

Veith I 1972 *Huang Ti Nei Ching Su Wen: The Yellow Emperor's Classic of Internal Medicine* (new edn). University of California, California

References

Anderson EM 1977 *The Golden Jubilee History 1923–1973: The New Zealand Association of Physiotherapists Inc*. The New Zealand Association of Physiotherapists Inc, Wellington

Australian Association of Massage Therapists (AAMT). Online. Available: http://www.aamt.com.au/ (accessed 1 Sept 2008)

Australian Massage Research Foundation (AMRF). Online. Available: http://www.amrf.org.au/ (accessed 1 Sept 2008)

Beard G, Wood EC 1964 *Massage Principles and Techniques*. W B Saunders, Philadelphia

Beck MF 1999 *Milady's Theory and Practice of Therapeutic Massage* (3rd edn). Milady, Albany

Bennett C 2003 Personal correspondence by email

Butler Colonel AG 1943 *The Official History of the Australian Army Medical Services in the War of 1914–1918, vol. 3*. Special Problems and Services. Australian War Memorial, Canberra

Calvert RN 2002 *The History of Massage — An Illustrated Survey From Around the World*. Healing Arts Press, Rochester, Vermont

Chandler CA 1980 Galen. *In: The World Book Encyclopedia* (vol 8). World Book-Childcraft International Inc, Chicago

Cyriax JH 1984 *Textbook of Orthopaedic Medicine: Volume 2* (11th edn). Baillière Tindall, London

Dunstan D, Bentley P (unpublished) 2000 *The Australian Physiotherapy Association Draft History*

Fay HJC 1912 *Scientific Massage for Athletes*. Ewart, Seymour & Co Ltd, Windsor House. Kingsway, London

HRH The Prince of Wales 2008 Reception to celebrate the formation of the Complementary and Natural Healthcare Council. 31 March

Kellogg JH 1895 *The Art of Massage: Its Physiological Effects and Therapeutic Applications*. Modern Medicine Publishing, Battle Creek, Michigan

Kleen EAG 1918 *Massage and Medical Gymnastics*. J & A Churchill, London

Massage New Zealand (MNZ). Online. Available: www.massagenewzealand.org (accessed 21 Oct 2009)

Martyr P 2002 *Paradise of Quacks, An Alternative History of Medicine in Australia*. Macleay Press, Sydney

McKay E 2002 *Touchline Magazine*. Queensland Association of Massage Therapists (QAMT), Brisbane

Mehta N 2000 *Indian Head Massage: Discover the Power of Touch*. Thorsons, UK

Mennell JB 1920 *Massage, Its Principles and Practice*. J & A Churchill, London

Palmer MD 1912 *Lessons on Massage* (4th edn). Baillière, Tindall and Cox, London

Peters A 1890 *Massage: Its History, Its Curative Uses, and Its Practical Results*. Public Library, Melbourne

Riley M 1994 *Maori Healing and Herbal*. Viking Sevenseas NZ Ltd, Paraparaumu

Salvo SG 1999 *Massage Therapy Principles and Practice*. W B Saunders, Philadelphia

Sanford J 2003 Personal correspondence by email

Smith C 1996 *ARM Massage Newsletter*. Association of Remedial Masseurs Incorporated (ARM)

Tall N 2003 Personal communication, 1 May

Tappan F 1988 *Healing Massage Techniques — Holistic, Classic and Emerging Methods* (2nd edn). Appleton & Lange, Connecticut

Unschuld PU 2000 *Medicine in China — Historical Artifacts and Images*. Prestel Verlag, Munich

Vautier B 2003 Personnel correspondence by email

Veith I 1972 *Huang Ti Nei Ching Su Wen: The Yellow Emperor's Classic of Internal Medicine* (new edn). University of California, California

Warren A 2003 Author's interview with Aboriginal elder from the Dtjilmamidtung region

Wittlinger H 2004 Emil Vodder — His Life and His Life's Work. Online. Available: www.vodderschool.com/-emil_vodder_life_work_article (accessed 16 Aug 2009)

massage in an integrative health care model
David Stelfox

chapter 3

LEARNING OUTCOMES

- **Define holistic health care**
- **Define integrative medicine**
- **Describe the benefits of massage therapy within an integrative approach to health care**

INTRODUCTION

Massage is as old as the art and science of healing itself. The majority of the cultures on this planet have incorporated bodywork, massage or manipulative therapy (i.e. physical manipulation of the body's muscles, ligaments, tendons and bones) within their traditional system of healing in some way. As outlined in Chapter 2, the earliest records of the use of massage date back over 3000 years and come from the East (Thailand and China). Other evidence suggests that over the centuries India, Tibet, Egypt, Polynesia, Indonesia, North and South America, Europe and Australia all have a history of the use of various forms of tactile therapy/bodywork within their healing traditions.

Each of these traditions recognised the benefits, indeed the necessity, of tactile therapy within its overall approach to health care. Furthermore, the indigenous healers from these cultures understood the importance of the health of mind, emotions, spirit and body, and their interrelatedness in regard to overall wellbeing. The therapies comprising these traditional healing systems were ones that aimed at specifically addressing each of these aspects of the health of a person — the mind, body, emotions and spirit.

While the techniques used or philosophies adopted may vary slightly from one culture to another, the modalities of therapy are indeed similar. Typically they include diet and nutrition therapy, the use of plant medicines (herbs), counselling (both psychological and spiritual), exercise therapy (e.g. yoga, tai qi, qi gong) and, of course, some form of tactile therapy/bodywork. Among indigenous people, massage or manipulative therapy was employed to exorcise evil spirits, to correct a person's physical structure or simply to make a person feel good. Ritual, prayer, devotion and often shamanic practice were also common features. Such practices have been passed down through generations of indigenous people, and continue to be used by many indigenous groups today.

WHAT IS HOLISTIC/INTEGRATIVE MEDICINE?

The word 'health' originally stems from the Germanic and Old English word hœlan meaning 'whole' (*Australian Concise Oxford Dictionary* 1995). The act of healing literally means the act of making whole, or restoring to a state of wholeness. Traditional medicine systems address each and every aspect of one's being, and as such are seen as 'holistic' or 'integrative' approaches. (W)Holistic medicine (the spelling differs for this word but the meaning is the same in either form) is an approach to health care that recognises the interconnectedness between the body, mind, emotions and spirit (i.e. it addresses the 'whole person').

The World Health Organization (WHO), a division of the United Nations, has defined holistic health care as (WHO 1998):

> that of viewing man in his totality within a wide ecological spectrum, and of emphasising the view that ill health or disease is brought about by an imbalance or disequilibrium of man in his total ecological system and not only by the causative agent and pathogenic evolution.

Furthermore, the WHO views traditional systems of health care as (WHO 1998):

> one of the surest means to achieve total health care coverage of the world's population, using safe and economically feasible methods.

'Integrative' medicine may be considered from two perspectives. The first perspective, similar to 'holistic' medicine, emphasises the unity, or integration, of mind, body, spirit and emotions in a healthy, balanced individual, and the use of appropriate therapies for attending to them. However, integrative medicine goes further than this, suggesting that the practitioners of these different therapies need to work cooperatively and in consultation with each other, as well as the client, so that health/wholeness and wellbeing can be optimally achieved and maintained. In this sense the various individual therapies within a medical system, and the practitioners of them, determine which therapies will be of greatest benefit to the patient/client at the time. Since they all work within the philosophical framework of that particular health system, and the principles that define it, then they have an understanding and appreciation of each of the therapies which comprise that system and recognise the value and importance of referral to specialist practitioners where necessary. The system of healing is therefore 'integrative' from this perspective.

Integrative therapies are sometimes administered by a single therapist who is skilled in the practice and theory of all of them. Sometimes it may be that a number of practitioners, each trained and skilled in a specialty area of treatment (e.g. bodywork/herbal medicine/counselling/exercise therapy/diet or nutrition) may work within an overall guiding philosophy of a particular healing system (e.g. traditional Chinese medicine/naturopathy/ayurveda).

The second perspective of integrative health care is a more contemporary one. Integrative health care is a term coined within the last 10 years by a new breed of general medical practitioner, one who recognises the value of integrating 'mainstream' biomedical health care with complementary/alternative/natural healing approaches. While this is an admirable view, it is often the case that such doctors (i.e. biomedical practitioners) have little understanding of the guiding philosophy/ies of the complementary healing approaches and the system of medicine they represent. It is perhaps a sad reflection of the current mainstream system of medicine that most of its practitioners are only prescribers of medicines. The integrative medicine approach, then, while appearing to integrate the best of both worlds, simply applies either 'mainstream' or 'alternative' medical approaches within the context of the Western biomedical model of health care. In such a model, natural medicine therapies are usually administered without regard to the philosophy or principles that define them (see Chapter 1), largely as alternatives to pharmaceutical drug therapy or, less commonly, surgery.

This approach is ultimately doomed to failure since it overlooks or simply dismisses the most beneficial features of the natural medicine health care model; that is, it's guiding principles — one of which is the concept of the doctor as teacher (*docere*). This principle stipulates that therapists should educate their clients and encourage self-responsibility for their health. It also recognises and promotes the therapeutic potential of the practitioner–client relationship. Any health care practitioner, whether of natural or orthodox medicine, who simply prescribes medications (natural or pharmaceutical) does the art of healing a great disservice.

INTEGRATIVE MEDICINE — THE HEALTH CARE MODEL FOR THE TWENTY-FIRST CENTURY

This chapter now examines the first perspective of integrative medicine (the one that considers the importance of body, mind, emotions and spirit for maintaining and restoring optimum health) and the role that massage therapy can play in delivering this unified approach to health care in the 21st century.

With the conscious recognition of the complexity of modern society there has emerged an awareness of the contributions of environment, lifestyle, stress, emotional disturbance, psychosocial and cultural factors and chronic 'unwellness' to the process of disease. As a result of this recognition, health care has begun to take a turn toward self-care, mind–body therapy, personal and spiritual development and wellness enhancement to counterbalance the excesses and limitations of the biomedical model (Dacher 2001). This turnaround is leading to a desire for a person-centred, wellness approach to health care rather than the disease-centred orientation that has characterised the Western biomedical model. The 21st century health care consumer demands to be seen as an individual whose experiences constitute a dynamic unity. Today's consumer holds a certain distrust or suspicion of most things perceived as 'scientific' (Siahpush 1998). The consumer demands an understanding of their existing health condition, and a desire to be actively involved in the process of improving that condition (Siahpush 1998). The appropriate health care model for this century must therefore cater to these consumer demands and provide choices based on patients' preferences, respect for other therapeutic approaches and acknowledgment of the specialised skills and expertise of practitioners of other therapies.

In other sections of this book, the value, indeed the importance, of touch in maintaining and promoting health is discussed at length. Massage, or any form of manual therapy that involves touch, inevitably impacts more than just the physical level of one's health. The idea of the body being touched in a deliberate way to achieve specific results is well documented and readily accepted, yet the ability of touch to evoke the powerful emotional responses and shifts in mental attitudes or spiritual perspective that often accompany most physical manipulations or tactile experiences is usually overlooked or ignored. Clearly, any integrative approach to healing must include massage or some other form of manipulative or tactile therapy. Let's now examine this claim in more detail.

MASSAGE AS COMPLEMENTARY THERAPY

The benefits of massage as an effective therapy in its own right must never be underestimated. However, this chapter will focus on the valuable contribution that massage has to make as a complement or adjunct to other approaches to healing — in other words, how it can augment the therapeutic value of other healing modalities.

Massage and naturopathy

Naturopathy incorporates an eclectic blend of therapies in its attempt to promote the body's ability to heal itself. Historically, manipulative therapy or massage has always been one of the healing modalities incorporated as part of this system of holistic health care (others include diet and nutrition therapy, herbal medicines, flower essences, homoeopathy, exercise, lifestyle counselling) (Lindlahr 1975). The main reason for the inclusion of massage or manipulative therapy is its ability to restore structural balance to the body while also helping to relieve stress and promote emotional, mental and spiritual wellbeing.

In Australia, 50% of practicing naturopaths incorporate massage in their practice (Hale 2002).This percentage is probably similar in New Zealand. In North America, naturopathy education programs include bodywork therapy, usually remedial massage and manipulative techniques. Similarly, in the UK naturopaths are trained in remedial massage techniques and employ them as an integral part of the naturopathic health care model. The inclusion of massage therapy as part of the naturopathic therapeutic strategy for a client can play a major role in helping to develop rapport between the practitioner and the client, and thereby enhance the healing potential of the client–practitioner relationship. The omission of massage from training courses in naturopathy has the potential to contribute to a trend towards 'prescription-pad medicine' (i.e. the prescribing of alternative drugs — herbs, nutritional supplements and homoeopathic remedies — without the inclusion of other important holistic considerations such as lifestyle counselling, dietary modification or any form of tactile therapy). The danger this presents is that the client is no longer the focus of attention. The client's symptoms and signs, and the disease, become the focus for treatment rather than the individual. This is something for which mainstream medical practitioners have been frequently criticised over the last 50 years.

In a world deprived of the benefits of touch, massage can provide nurturing and comfort to many people (Johnson 1985; see also Chapter 4). When so many of the health problems experienced today stem from the stress and emotional confusion associated with 21st century living, tactile therapy provides a means by which unexpressed or suppressed emotions such as grief, sadness, anger and frustration might be safely released. It is well known that emotions such as these are a common part of the experience of most physical illness (even having the effect of further compounding and complicating the disease picture). Therefore massage is clearly an important part of the naturopath's treatment strategy as a holistic practitioner.

Part of the process for delivering a massage or tactile therapy treatment requires provision of a suitable environment — that is, a healing environment. A healing environment is one that cocoons the client, and the therapist, from the outside world. It provides security, comfort, serenity and a feeling of being nurtured. In such an environment the client feels safe to contemplate the nature of their disease; to ponder the causes or contributing factors. It is a healing space; something hard to find in the often chaotic world of today. In such a space, it is possible that the individual can discover what may be required of them to obtain a satisfactory improvement of, if not a resolution to, their health problems. The naturopath must be aware of this potential and seek to provide her/his clients with this opportunity whenever appropriate.

On the physiological level, one of the many benefits of massage therapy is to improve circulation throughout the tissues of the body. This circulation is not restricted to the blood, but also includes lymph, interstitial and intracellular fluids. It may also extend to the circulation of energy or vital force. In many healing traditions massage and soft tissue manipulation were employed primarily to remove obstacles and promote the unimpeded flow of life energy (e.g. Qi or Prana) via the subtle energy channels or meridians.

Nutrients, oxygen, hormones, antibodies and other immunisers, and of course water, must be delivered to every single cell continually if it is to survive and respond the way it should, and all kinds of toxic wastes must be borne away. There is no tissue that cannot be weakened and ultimately destroyed by chronic interruptions of these various circulations (Juhan 1998).

Kaptchuk and Croucher in their book *The Healing Arts — A Journey Through the Faces of Medicine* (1986) make the following comment (p 38) concerning the omission of tactile therapy from the practice of medicine:

> Perhaps the greatest loss that medicine has suffered over the course of the centuries is that of personal contact. Sophisticated doctors throughout the world tend to avoid the healing power of the human hand. The only form of contact that seems to have survived worldwide is the elevated art of surgery — perhaps because it can be practised in the most detached and impersonal setting. Other types of physical contact are dispersed into secondary, often disparaged categories, which are left to vie among themselves for some badge of accomplishment: osteopathy, chiropractic, acupuncture, bonesetting and manipulation and massage in its many forms.
>
> Far from being able to exude a feeling of fellowship and warmth, in many societies, doctors, especially men, have assumed the mantle of an unapproachable priesthood. Worse, the profession condemns some, and discourages many, of the therapies of touch that have helped millions of people physically as well as psychologically. From the perspective of other cultures and other times such attitudes could politely be described as provincial.

Naturopaths must be careful that they do not make this same mistake and view massage as a form of second-rate manual labour, discarding it from their therapeutic repertoire in favour of the glamour and appeal of 'prescription-pad medicine'. Without the inclusion of massage as a therapy, naturopathy would struggle to address emotional, mental and spiritual aspects of health and perhaps fail in its effort to provide true holistic, integrative health care.

Massage and acupuncture

The same can be said of acupuncture, or traditional Chinese medicine (TCM), as has been stated for naturopathy. Without the inclusion of tactile therapy, acupuncture is a therapeutic modality, not a holistic system of health care. Thankfully, the practice of acupuncture involves making physical contact, but this contact may be brief, and may be administered with clinical efficiency rather than in a way that is comforting and nurturing. Similarly, the inclusion of an mo tui na (traditional Chinese massage) in the TCM system (of which acupuncture is a part) focuses largely on achieving a therapeutic result, and the techniques employed are often strong, forceful and dynamic. While the Western approach to massage therapy (e.g. Swedish style) was derived originally from the Chinese an mo tui na, it is generally less forceful, as pain is considered undesirable in the Western world.

The inclusion of a more gentle approach to massage in a TCM or acupuncture practice may offer many benefits to the Western client. This is certainly not suggesting that Chinese massage therapy is in any way less effective — simply that the Western mind/psyche may respond more readily to an approach that is perceived as gentler, more soothing, more comforting and more relaxing. The impact of such an approach on the emotional, mental and spiritual wellbeing of a client may be more successful than a more forceful one, and from this perspective is certainly worth considering as an adjunct to acupuncture and TCM.

Massage and homoeopathy

A typical homoeopathic consultation involves extensive case-taking on the part of the practitioner. The client undergoes a thorough interview process during which many details concerning the individual's health, symptoms and signs, personality and likes and dislikes are determined so that the most appropriate homoeopathic remedy can be determined and prescribed according to the indications. While the process is most extensive, and calls upon the client to consider issues that are physical, emotional, mental and spiritual, the interview process may be seen as very much a cerebral exercise.

The incorporation of massage as part of the treatment package for homoeopathy can certainly add another dimension to the treatment experience. As previously discussed, the benefits of tactile therapy in contributing to the client–practitioner relationship, and the contribution of that relationship to the healing process, are quite significant. The contribution of the client–practitioner relationship to the process of healing has been estimated to be at least 40%. Thirty-five per cent of the process of healing is attributed to 'self-healing' and

25% is attributed to the actual therapy employed (Miller 1998). The positive experience of a massage treatment when combined with a homoeopathic prescription can only produce a therapeutic outcome with more impact for the client.

Massage and osteopathy, chiropractic and physiotherapy

It is becoming increasingly commonplace for massage therapists to work together with other manipulative therapists (i.e. osteopaths, chiropractors and physiotherapists) for the purpose of achieving optimum results with musculoskeletal health problems. While there has been a significant movement away from high velocity–low amplitude (HVLA) thrusting adjustments (Chaitow 2001) resulting in a number of chiropractors, osteopaths and physiotherapists adopting much gentler manipulations of the soft tissues of the body, a large number of these practitioners still focus predominantly on spinal adjustments. Massage complements this type of work, especially when it is administered prior to a high-speed manipulative treatment, by relaxing the muscles and nervous system, and improving circulation to the problem areas. In achieving this, the client is effectively prepared for the treatment that will follow.

Often, as a result of tight or hypertonic muscles, it may be difficult for a manipulative therapist to achieve a satisfactory result for a client without some preliminary soft tissue work being performed. Furthermore, regular appropriate massage may be beneficial as ongoing therapy, both to maintain the results of the manipulative therapy and also to possibly reduce the need for excessive follow-up treatment.

It is important for massage therapists to recognise the scope of their knowledge and skills, to develop professional relationships with other health care providers, including chiropractors, osteopaths and physiotherapists, and to feel comfortable to refer their clients to other therapists who may be able to better address the health needs of the client. As massage therapists and practitioners of the other various manipulative therapies see the positive results of working together cooperatively, either in their separate or in integrated practices, they feel more confident and comfortable with such an arrangement and their clientele spreads word of their satisfaction. Trust and effective communication are no doubt key factors to a successful integrative practice, and to working towards achieving what is best for the client.

Massage and fitness therapy, personal training and sports coaching

While the benefit of massage therapy to sporting performance is well established, its application to fitness therapy and personal training is perhaps a little less obvious.

For decades coaches of all sports have called upon the massage therapist to prepare their sportsmen and women for optimum performance, to help them recover from the trauma of the event and from physical injury.

Massage therapists now accompany most professional sporting teams and the number of massage therapists who provide their services at the Olympic games has increased significantly every 4 years. With the ever-increasing commercialisation of sport and the associated pressure on sportsmen and women to succeed, the inclusion of the massage therapist as a crucial member of the team is obviously essential. It seems certain that the demand for well-trained, competent massage therapists who specialise in sports massage will continue to increase.

Personal trainers and fitness therapists primarily focus on improving the level of fitness, strength and flexibility of their clients. Demand for the services of these professionals has increased markedly as a result of the trend towards improved physical health and well-being, and the desire to look and feel vital and youthful. These professionals work as consultants, providing advice and direction, and prescribing exercise regimens to achieve the desired result for the client. Some assist in the prevention of, and recovery from, injury. It makes perfect sense then for these trainers/therapists to offer the services of massage therapy to their clients to augment the training programs they recommend. Regular massage may speed the process of recovery from rigorous training sessions and promote optimum musculoskeletal function so that clients will get more out of their exercise schedules.

MASSAGE AND THE BIOMEDICAL MODEL OF HEALTH CARE

It seems strange when every other culture on the planet has included massage therapy in its traditional system of medicine that Western society chose in the past to abandon, and even discourage, the use of it for healing. A brief look at the history of Western medicine seems to indicate that the exclusion of massage therapy from that system had more to do with tradition than with reason.

Dr Johann Mezger, the Dutch physician (see Chapter 2), established massage as a credible part of mainstream medical practice in the mid-19th century. Its use then spread throughout Europe with such famous physicians as Lucas-Championnière and Charcot, in France, promoting its use. Lucas-Championnière published the textbook *Massage and Mobilisation in the Treatment of Fractures* for the use of fellow physicians (Lucas-Championnière 1895). But by the late 1800s, doctors in Britain were already expressing an unwillingness to administer such a manual procedure themselves, and were advocating the training of nurses (female) to deliver massage treatments, under their close supervision, in the hospitals.

It seems that this led to an increase in the popularity and demand for massage and women other than nurses undertook private training in the art of massage. Seeing such unsupervised practice as a threat to their own livelihood and status as healers, British doctors issued a warning, via *The British Medical Journal* (1894), against young women training in massage as a career. The article stated (p 88) that there was no demand for

masseuses and also warned against the unsavoury nature of massage as practised in some so-called massage establishments in London. Surgery's significant rise in status had a lot to do with the decline in use of massage and manipulative therapy by physicians. Relegated to the lowly status of barbers during the Middle Ages, surgeons were previously regarded as relatively unskilled and their 'art' was seen as a last-resort approach.

'Surgery' derives from the Greek word meaning 'hand work'. Physicians were once seen as superior to surgeons in terms of their training, knowledge and skills, and were therefore given the title of 'Doctor' (teacher) to reflect their elevated status. Surgeons, on the other hand, were manual, hands-on practitioners who were also trained as barbers (barber–surgeons). They held the title of 'Mister' which reflected their lower status. These titles are maintained today, although the status attached to each is a reversal of the previous.

While the use of massage in hospitals continued at a low level throughout the Western world during the early 20th century (mainly due to the efforts of nurses who saw the benefits it offered to patients), its popularity within the Western system of medicine dwindled as a direct result of distrust and dissuasion of its use by doctors (Martyr 2002).

The development of the pharmaceutical industry and the associated fascination with the potential of the 'magic bullet' (miracle drugs) was another factor. It wasn't until the 1960s when physiotherapy became a registered profession, that massage or manipulative therapy regained any sort of approval from the orthodox medical profession.

The 1970s saw the recognition of massage's value as part of a holistic approach to health care. Its increase in popularity outside of the orthodox health system brought about greater general interest and enquiry. Early research explored its potential for enhancing health. With more research, and greater awareness of its many benefits, renewed interest in the inclusion of massage in mainstream health care is occurring. Nursing homes and some private hospitals have introduced massage therapy as a form of complementary care. While there is still considerable resistance from some doctors and hospital administrators, support for massage therapy's inclusion in the mainstream medical system is substantial. It seems certain that before long the doors will open and tactile therapies, including massage, will be seen as another branch of orthodox medical care.

In the USA, therapeutic touch (a subtle energy approach to healing) is widely administered by nurses to patients in hospital settings. Therapeutic touch, developed by nurses for nurses, stemmed from the realisation that hospital patients were usually touch deprived and that their recovery could be significantly enhanced through some form of tactile therapy. Nurses are ideally suited to delivering tactile therapy to patients in hospital wards, as they are familiar with the patient's health condition, his or her personal likes and dislikes, and have (in most cases) gained the patient's trust and acceptance.

At a time when hospital budgets are severely restricted and nurses struggle to deliver even the basic services to patients due to time and staffing constraints, it seems unlikely that tactile therapy in any form (e.g. relaxation massage, reiki, touch for health, remedial massage) will become commonplace in public hospitals. However, some hospitals have introduced massage services to patients, and experience suggests that the outcomes (in terms of patient wellbeing and recovery) are positive. More research (in particular, clinical trials) is needed to explore the potential benefits of massage or other tactile therapy in the hospital wards. It is only as a result of positive research findings that authorities may be willing to examine the possibility of providing massage therapy (whether for relaxation or remedial purposes) to hospital patients.

The prospect of massage therapy being performed prior to and after surgery, as an adjunct to the process of recovery, is an inspiring one. However, it is not an original notion. In the fourteenth century the esteemed French physician Guy de Chauliac published a book on surgical procedure, *Inventorium sive collectorium in parte chirurgiciali medicin*. It became a standard text throughout Europe for the next 200 years. The book described the administration of various methods of massage and manipulation to augment surgical procedures.

WHY PEOPLE USE MASSAGE THERAPY

In a 2002 national survey on Americans' use of complementary and alternative medicine (CAM), respondents who used a CAM therapy could choose from five reasons for using the therapy. The results for massage were as follows:

1   They believed that massage combined with conventional medicine would help: 60%
2   They thought massage would be interesting to try: 44%
3   They believed that conventional medical treatments would not help: 34%
4   Massage was suggested by a conventional medical professional: 33%
5   They thought that conventional medicine was too expensive: 13%

(Barnes et al 2004)

These survey results indicate that the majority of US consumers of massage therapy believe that the integration of conventional medical treatment with massage therapy is helpful. The results also indicate that a significant number of conventional medical practitioners suggested or recommended massage therapy to their patients.

In a 2004 New Zealand study, 74% (55) of general practitioners surveyed stated that they had recommended patients to see a massage therapist in the past 12 months (Lawler & Cameron 2004). A 2005 Australian study, which surveyed general practitioners' (GPs') attitudes toward complementary therapies, found that most Australian GPs regarded massage therapy as highly effective and safe and that GPs were willing to recommend massage for their patients (Cohen et al 2005).

Similar studies in the UK and Canada also suggest an increase in GPs' acceptance and confidence in referring patients for complementary therapies including massage (Marwick 2003).

With advances in scientific understanding, and as more is learnt about how the human organism functions, massage and manipulation therapy is once again emerging as a legitimate and desirable (perhaps essential) health care modality. Its inclusion in the mainstream biomedical health care model is inevitable. How long this will take is perhaps the only uncertainty.

According to sociological surveys, Australians are no longer satisfied with the system of health care they have been offered to date (Siahpush 1998). To satisfy the demands of the Australian public it is clear that an integrative model of health care is necessary.

CONCLUSION

An integrative model is one that provides choice in the range of therapeutic options it can offer. It also provides an approach that views the human being as a unity of body, mind, emotions and spirit, and appreciates the need for addressing each of these aspects as a means of promoting, restoring and maintaining optimum health.

Massage therapy has a vital role to play as part of an integrative model of health care. It complements the benefits of other therapeutic modalities and, in itself, has positive benefits for each of the four aspects of health (i.e. body, mind, emotions and spirit). These benefits have been established empirically due to the inclusion of massage therapy in the majority of traditional systems of healing as practised by the indigenous people of the planet's many cultures.

An integrative system of medicine also requires that the practitioners of the various therapies that comprise it are broad-minded and tolerant of each other's principles and philosophies. Furthermore, they must have a general understanding and appreciation of how other therapies work and what they are attempting to achieve. Massage therapists therefore must be prepared to study the basic principles of other healing modalities — those that comprise what is currently described as the Western biomedical or mainstream approach to medicine, as well as those that comprise the natural therapies approach. This is in no way to suggest that massage therapists who gain a broad understanding of other healing modalities or health care approaches should attempt to practice them or to incorporate them in their clinic, without gaining a full qualification in any of those modalities. Working outside of one's scope of practice is risky and may result in negligent practice that causes harm to the client.

A willingness to work cooperatively with therapists of other modalities, to refer when necessary, and to always place the interests of the client first — these are the other requirements of an integrative approach to healing.